(Hons). She was deputy cookery editor on ░░░░░░░░░░ ly magazine and later cookery editor of *Home*. ░░░░░░ ░w a full-time writer and food consultant to various lifestyle and health magazines and has written more than sixty cookbooks. She specialises in healthy eating, and her recent published books include *The Vegan Dairy* and *Gluten-Free Kitchen* and *Fermenting Foods for Healthy Eating*.

ALSO BY CATHERINE ATKINSON

Brilliant Breadmaking in Your Bread Machine
Cooking with Your Instant Pot
Fermenting Food for Healthy Eating
Gluten-Free Kitchen
Healthy Meals for Healthy Kids
How to Make Perfect Panini
How to Make Your Own Cordials and Syrups
Power Blends and Smoothies
The Spiralizer Cookbook
The Vegan Dairy

The Healthy Fibre-Rich Cookbook

Recipes to Increase Your Fibre Intake and Help You Feel Fantastic

Catherine Atkinson

A HOW TO BOOK

ROBINSON

ROBINSON

First published in Great Britain in 2021 by Robinson

10 9 8 7 6 5 4 3 2 1

A CIP catalogue record for this book is available from the British Library.

ISBN: 978-1-47214-577-2

Typeset by Basement Press, Glaisdale
Printed and bound in Great Britain by Clays Ltd, Elcograf S.p.A.

Papers used by Robinson are from well-managed forests and other responsible sources.

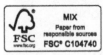

MIX
Paper from
responsible sources
FSC® C104740

Robinson
An imprint of
Little, Brown Book Group
Carmelite House
50 Victoria Embankment
London EC4Y 0DZ

An Hachette UK Company
www.hachette.co.uk

www.littlebrown.co.uk

How To Books are published by Robinson, an imprint of Little, Brown Book Group. We welcome proposals from authors who have first-hand experience of their subjects. Please set out the aims of your book, its target market and its suggested contents in an email to howtobooks@littlebrown.co.uk

Note on the recipes
Unless otherwise stated, vegetable and egg sizes are medium; vegetables are trimmed and peeled as necessary.

Contents

Introduction **1**

Fibre Facts **3**

Basic Preparation for your Store Cupboard **23**

Breakfasts and Brunches **27**
    Crunchy Granola Cereal **28**
    Quinoa Berry Porridge **30**
    Overnight Oats **32**
    Buttermilk Banana Pancakes **34**
    Apricot Spread **36**
    Dried Fruit Compote **38**
    Oat and Bran Honey Muffins **40**
    Breakfast Bars **42**
    Pear and Raspberry Smoothie **44**
    Lower-Fat Eggs Benedict **46**

Soups, Salads and Snacks **49**
    Chunky Vegetable and Lentil Soup **50**
    Green Pea and Flageolet Bean Soup
      with Minted Yogurt **52**
    Chicken Noodle Soup **54**
    Classic Minestrone **56**
    Roasted Red Pepper and Tomato Soup **58**
    Chicken Satay Wraps **60**
    Chickpea Scotch Eggs **62**
    Dips and Dippers (hummus, avocado and
      watercress dip, vegetable crudités) **64**
    Baked Vegetable Crisps and Tortilla Chips **66**
    Warm Prawn, Avocado and Wholewheat
      Couscous Salad **68**
    Oriental Sprouted Salad **70**
    Turkey and Cranberry Salad with Barley **72**
    Lighter Nachos **74**

Upside-Down Pizza **76**
Mini Pizza Grills **78**
Baked Spanish Omelette **80**
Re-Fried Bean Burritos with Fresh Tomato Salsa **82**
Feta, Black-Eyed Bean and Potato Parcels **84**
Classic Kimchi **86**
Quinoa Falafels in Wholemeal Pittas **88**

Main Meals **91**

Moroccan-Style Chicken and Chickpea Casserole **92**
Creamy Chicken, Mushroom and Artichoke Filo Pie **94**
One-Pan Roast Chicken with Vegetables **96**
Cheese-Topped Chicken and Mushroom Enchiladas **98**
Turkey Meatballs in Tomato Sauce **100**
Chinese-Spiced Duck and Kumquats **102**
Duck and Mixed Mushroom Risotto **104**
Beef Jambalaya **106**
Updated Cottage Pie **108**
Mediterranean Lamb and Vegetable Kebabs **110**
Lamb Tagine **112**
Sweet and Spicy Stir-Fried Pork **114**
Smoked Salmon and Asparagus Quiche with a Spelt
    and Sesame Crust **116**
Glazed Cod with Fresh Tomato Dressing **118**
Melting-Middle Fishcakes **120**
Fresh Tuna Niçoise **122**
Cauliflower and Chickpea Burgers **124**
Goat's Cheese and Lentil Loaf **126**
Cheese and Potato Slice **128**
Vegetable Tikka Masala **130**

Desserts **133**

No-Bake Blueberry Cheesecake **134**
Banana Rice Pudding **136**
Oaty Apricot Crumble **138**
Sticky Toffee Puddings **140**
Cherry Bakewell Sponge **142**
Pumpkin Pie **144**

Raspberry and Rose Frozen Yogurt **146**
Chocolate and Coconut Ice Cream **148**
Peaches and Cream Winter Fool **150**
Pineapple and Orange Jelly **152**
Fresh Fig Compote **154**
Chocolate and Avocado Mousse **156**

Baking **159**

Sweet Potato Bread Rolls **160**
Multi-Grain Bread **162**
Sun-Dried Tomato and Olive Focaccia **164**
Butternut Squash Cornbread **166**
Cheddar and Watercress Scones **168**
Banana and Date Loaf **170**
Tropical Fruit Malt Teabread **172**
Carrot and Coconut Cake **174**
Chocolate Chunk Black-Bean Brownies **176**
Oat and Apple Cookies **178**
Peanut Butter Cookies **180**
Wholemeal Spelt and Honey Biscuits **182**
Digestive Biscuits **184**
Cheese and Seed Oatcakes **186**

Conversion Charts **188**

Index **191**

INTRODUCTION

So much has been written in the past decade about what we should and shouldn't eat that it's hard to know what dietary advice to follow. One message has always been loud and clear: we should all be eating more dietary fibre. We know that fibre helps to keep our digestive systems healthy, but not everyone knows that a fibre-rich diet can reduce blood sugar and cholesterol levels, it also helps to control weight and reduces the risk of developing heart disease, type-2 diabetes and certain cancers. UK guidelines say that our intake of dietary fibre should increase to around 30g a day as part of a healthy balanced diet, yet most adults are eating less than half this amount.

With advances in technology and food production, an increasing choice of foods is available, yet most of us eat a more limited range than our ancestors. Many modern diets are low in fibre and instead are packed with processed foods, refined carbohydrates and sugar.

A fibre-rich diet is not a new trend and was popular in the 1980s. Fibre was then often labelled 'roughage'. Synonymous with bran, it was often thought of simply as a bulking agent. Nutritional knowledge has evolved since then and we now know that dietary fibre has many more benefits and plays a vital role in a balanced diet. Dietitians no longer advise people to eat lots of bran-based cereals, and we are now encouraged to eat more fruit and vegetables – at least five portions daily, and preferably more.

This book includes the most recent developments and nutritional knowledge about fibre. There is no need to buy a whole range of specialist ingredients; it's more about adjusting your meals and eating habits and making a few simple changes, which can be introduced over time. Here, I will show you why you should eat more fibre and how easy it is to incorporate it into your everyday diet. You will also find a range of up-to-date recipes to suit everyone and to inspire you on your journey to better health.

FIBRE FACTS

The role of dietary fibre in a healthy, balanced diet should not be underestimated. It is obtained solely from foods of plant origin and there are two kinds. They are of equal importance, although nutritionists now worry less about distinguishing between the two, as most plants contain both types but in differing proportions; for example, the fibre content of an avocado (Hass variety) contains about 63 per cent insoluble fibre and 37 per cent soluble fibre.

Insoluble fibre absorbs water and bulks up the food in our gut so that it keeps it moving smoothly through the digestive tract. This is the type that used to be referred to as roughage.

Soluble fibre slows down the breakdown of complex carbohydrates, such as starch, into simple sugars such as glucose, helping to keep blood sugar levels stable. It can lower levels of the harmful kind of cholesterol, because during digestion it forms a gel-like mass that binds cholesterol and removes it from the body.

Sources of insoluble and soluble fibre

INSOLUBLE

Plant source	Examples
Wheat	Wholemeal bread, flour and pastas; wheat bran
Maize	Sweetcorn, polenta (cornmeal)
Rice	Brown rice and brown rice flour
Fruit	Berries (strawberries, raspberries, etc.), rhubarb
Leafy vegetables	Cabbage, kale, spinach, lettuce
Pulses	Dried beans, peas, chickpeas, lentils

SOLUBLE

Plant source	Examples
Oats	Porridge, muesli
Barley	Pearl and pot barley
Rye	Rye bread, rye crispbread
Fruit	Apples, apricots, figs, tomatoes
Root and vine vegetables	Carrots, potatoes, parsnips, courgettes
Pulses	Baked beans, kidney beans, black beans

FIBRE FOR HEALTH

Vital to our health and well-being, dietary fibre can help digestion, prevent constipation and make you feel fuller for longer. It also plays an important role in helping to prevent and to fight disease and illnesses. Eating plenty of fibre can reduce the risk of heart attack and stroke, certain cancers, including bowel cancer, and type-2 diabetes. Because fibre boosts the level of short-chain fatty acids produced by bacteria in the gut, it plays an important role in the health of joints and bones, helping to lower the risk of inflammatory diseases such as rheumatoid arthritis and osteoporosis. As current research continues, it is likely that scientists might uncover further benefits of fibre.

KEEPING THINGS MOVING

Mention a fibre-rich diet and the first comments you are likely to hear are about bowel motions and constipation. It is a subject people either talk about with great amusement or refuse to discuss at all. Constipation is defined as passing bowel motions less frequently than twice a week or straining to do so more than 25 per cent of the time. Although it has many possible causes, the most common is not eating enough fibre. Bowel habits can vary between individuals, and it's perfectly normal to go once or several times a day, every other day or even less often, but if you experience a change in your routine, or it becomes difficult to pass stools and they are hard, dry, or abnormally large or small, you are suffering from constipation.

A fibre-rich diet helps to prevent constipation and ensures regular bowel movements. Stimulant laxatives should be a last and temporary resort (unless prescribed) and should never be used as a dieting aid, as they can make the intestine sensitive to their effects.

If you suffer from constipation, it is important to increase your fluid intake and you should aim to drink at least 1.2 litres (six 200ml glasses) a day, but limit alcohol and caffeinated drinks as they can lead to dehydration.

Magnesium can help to loosen stools, so choose some fibre-rich foods which are also a good source of magnesium, such as beans and pulses, almonds, Brazil nuts, cashew nuts, peanuts, raisins, sunflower and sesame seeds, spinach and artichokes. All these have at least 50mg of magnesium per 100g. A persistent change in bowel habit, especially in someone over the age of forty, should always be reported to a doctor to rule out the possibility of a more serious underlying factor.

GETTING TO KNOW YOUR GUT

Your body is home to an army of trillions of beneficial bacteria, which keep harmful bacteria under control and help us to fight infections. There are at least four hundred different species, which live naturally inside your gut, and they need to be looked after. Although research is still in its early days, we now know that it is vital to maintain a good balance of gut bacteria. As well as aiding digestion and assimilation, and absorption of nutrients, bacteria nourish the cells of the gut wall, keeping it healthy, and they produce important vitamins, minerals and chemicals. One of these is serotonin, which is involved in mood, hence the expression 'gut feelings'. Beneficial bacteria help to strengthen immunity by crowding out pathogenic (harmful) bacteria, such as those which cause strep throat and food poisoning, and yeasts such as candida and provide health-supporting probiotics to make your immune system more robust.

Fibre is fermented in the large intestine by gut bacteria to produce short-chain fatty acids. These are a major source of energy for the cells that line the colon, keeping it healthy. Short-chain fatty acids reduce the risk of inflammatory diseases and can also help to maintain weight, as they are involved in regulating fat metabolism by increasing fat burning and decreasing fat storage. When the intestines contain a balance of good and bad bacteria necessary for good health, they are described as being in a state of symbiosis. When this process is disrupted, it is known as 'dysbiosis', an imbalance in the gut microbiome caused by too few beneficial bacteria and an overgrowth of bad bacteria and yeasts. If you are unwell and need a course of antibiotics, most of the beneficial gut bacteria might be wiped out, leaving you with a weak immune system and susceptible to illness; however, it's not all doom and gloom: by eating a more varied diet and including plenty of fibre-rich foods, you can start to boost the diversity and number of beneficial gut bacteria in just a few days.

Boosting beneficial bacteria in the gut

Diversity matters because there are thousands of plant phytochemicals that are thought to feed different bacteria. It is important to eat as many different sources of fibre as possible. Bacteria in the large intestine quickly adapt to the types of fibre in your diet, so if you consistently eat fibre from just one or two sources for more than a week or two, bacteria will respond by increasing the enzymes needed to ferment this. This means that fibre reaching your colon will then be broken down faster and some of the benefits might be lost. Start by including fibre-rich foods that already contain beneficial bacteria: onions, garlic, asparagus and bananas are good sources. Even if you love routine, try to eat different fruit on different days. If you eat porridge every day, vary the toppings and have sliced bananas one day, and mixed berries or seeds or nuts the next. You should also aim to add more resistant starch to your diet (these are carbohydrates that resist digestion in the small intestine and ferment in the large intestine). There are high levels in lentils, seeds, brown rice, wholewheat pasta and potatoes.

AVOIDING DIVERTICULAR DISORDER

Diverticulosis is the presence of small pouches (diverticuli) in the wall of the colon. These occur when parts of the intestine bulge outwards through weak areas. The increase in pressure in the colon is often caused by constipation. Preventing and treating diverticulosis usually just involves increasing the amount of insoluble fibre in the diet together with plenty of fluids. This is particularly important if you already have diverticulosis, as straining when you go to the toilet will cause more diverticuli to form, and symptoms including cramps, bloating and irregular bowel movements will worsen.

Occasionally, the diverticuli might become inflamed and infected; this is known as diverticulitis. This occurs when a stool gets trapped in one of the pouches. The symptoms are more severe and include abdominal pain, nausea and fever. When this occurs the nutritional advice changes and for a short time you need to reduce fibre intake and follow a 'soft' diet that requires little or no chewing, such as soup, mashed potatoes and mashed bananas. Once the infection has cleared, the diet should revert to one that is rich in fibre.

TREATING IRRITABLE BOWEL SYNDROME (IBS)

IBS is a relatively common condition that affects the gut, causing intermittent abdominal discomfort and bloating often accompanied by either constipation or diarrhoea. During periods of constipation, relieve IBS by eating as many different sources of fibre as possible, including complex (unrefined) carbohydrates such as wholegrain bread and unsweetened wholegrain breakfast cereals. Soluble fibre such as that found in oats, ground flax seeds (linseeds), peeled potatoes and carrots are particularly helpful. During bouts of diarrhoea, eat a lower-fibre diet for a few days.

Many who have IBS find that particular foods trigger their symptoms. This varies hugely between individuals, so it is useful to keep a food diary and discover which, if any, foods cause flare-ups.

Many people find that dairy products such as milk are difficult to tolerate due to the lactose (the sugar in milk) content, but do not rule out yogurt; this is usually tolerated and contains beneficial bacteria, which supply lactase, the enzyme needed to digest lactose, as well as being a great source of calcium.

Some find that they need to limit fruit to a maximum of three 80g portions a day and avoid drinking fruit juice or fruit teas, as these contain a lot of fructose, which might aggravate symptoms.

Others find that they should steer clear of large servings of vegetables that are more difficult to digest, such as onions, cabbage, cauliflower, broccoli and Brussels sprouts. It is important to find out if such foods are triggers for you, rather than limiting your diet unnecessarily, so ask your doctor to refer you to a nutritionist or specialist.

PREVENTING GALLSTONES

The gallbladder is a small pouch-like organ situated underneath the liver. Its main purpose is to store and concentrate bile, which is produced by the liver to help digest fats. When levels of cholesterol in the bile become too high, the excess forms into 'stones'. These are very common and at least 10 per cent of adults in the UK have gallstones, although only a small number of these develop symptoms. The most at-risk group is obese women over the age of forty. If a gallstone blocks one of the bile ducts, it causes sudden and severe abdominal pain, which might last for several hours.

Avoiding fatty foods and increasing your consumption of fibre can help to prevent gallstones from developing and relieve the discomfort caused by existing stones. If you are obese, you are at increased risk of developing gallstones and should aim to lose weight; however, this should be gradual, as rapid weight loss can cause the formation of gallstones in some people.

STOPPING THE DEVELOPMENT OF TYPE-2 DIABETES

Over twelve million people in the UK are at risk of developing type-2 diabetes. A raised blood sugar level occurs when the body's ability to control glucose levels is impaired. This usually results from decreased production of the hormone insulin in the pancreas (type-1 diabetes) or from reduced sensitivity of body cells to the effects of insulin (type-2 diabetes). Nothing can be done to prevent type-1 diabetes and, whereas factors such as your age, ethnicity and family history all contribute towards your overall risk, around three in five cases of type-2 diabetes can be prevented or delayed by maintaining a healthy weight (see page 12), being active and eating well. Eating refined carbohydrates (white bread, white rice and sugary breakfast cereals) is linked with an increased risk of type-2 diabetes, whereas adding just two servings of wholegrain products each day can lower your risk by as much as 20 per cent. You should increase the amount of fruit and vegetables in your diet (there's no need to cut down on natural sugar that occurs in whole fruit). Certain fruit and vegetables are specifically associated with a reduced risk. These include apples, berries, grapes and green leafy vegetables such as kale, watercress, rocket and spinach.

If you have diabetes, both types of dietary fibre, but particularly soluble fibre can help to slow the absorption of sugar and improve blood sugar levels.

DECREASING THE RISKS OF CANCER

The World Cancer Research Fund has estimated that by eating a balanced diet including plenty of fibre-rich fruit and vegetables, whole grains and pulses, together with maintaining a healthy weight, as many as a third of all cancer deaths could be prevented.

Fruit and vegetables contain many vitamins, minerals and phytochemicals, which have an antioxidant effect that protects cells from cancer. There are hundreds of different phytochemicals. They are all protective chemicals, but a handful are of particular interest in helping to protect against cancer.

PROTECTIVE PHYTOCHEMICALS

Phytochemical	Good food sources	Protection
Glucosinolates	Broccoli, cabbage, cauliflower, kale	May prevent tumour growth, particularly in breast, lung, liver, stomach and colon cancer
Phytoestrogens	Soya products and flax seeds (linseeds)	May help slow the progression of certain cancers such as breast cancer
Indoles	Broccoli, pak choi, cabbage, turnip	May prevent breast cancer
Lycopene	Tomato, red pepper, pink grapefruit, papaya, mango and watermelon	Helps protect against prostate, cervix, stomach, bladder and colon cancer
Para-coumaric acid	Barley, peanuts, carrot, garlic and tomato	Interferes with the development of cancer-causing nitrosamines in the stomach
Terpenes	Apples, mango, citrus fruit, herbs and spices such as basil, rosemary and cinnamon	May block carcinogens, which could inhibit hormone-related cancers such as ovarian cancer

Fibre can help to eliminate cancer-related toxins and it also helps the body to eradicate free radicals. These are chemical by-products generated during normal biochemical reactions in the body. Highly reactive, they are needed to destroy bacteria, fight inflammation and maintain muscles. When they have fulfilled their purpose, it is important for the body to eliminate them. If they build up, free radicals can cause damage to the body's cells and tissues in a process known as oxidation.

Whole grains and flax seeds (linseeds) are a good source of some of the B-vitamins and compounds known as lignans, and these are thought to have a protective role against breast, prostate and colorectal cancers.

Being overweight increases your risk of developing cancer because fat cells produce extra growth hormones, which make the cells in our body divide more often. This increases the chance of cancer cells being produced. Excess weight increases the risk of getting bowel, uterus, oesophagus, pancreas, kidney, liver, stomach, gall bladder, thyroid and (in women after the menopause) breast cancers, as well as meningioma (a type of brain tumour) and myeloma (a type of blood cancer). A fibre-rich diet can help you to lose excess weight (see page 12) and maintain it.

LOWERING THE RISK OF CARDIOVASCULAR DISEASE AND STROKE

It is estimated that one in three deaths from coronary heart disease or stroke are due to an unhealthy diet. Although a cardio-protective diet is complex, the vital role of fibre is thought to stem from its ability to lower both blood pressure and cholesterol. A diet rich in fibre has been shown to reduce levels of low-density lipoproteins (LDL – the 'bad' cholesterol) by about 5 per cent.

Furthermore, eating foods which are high in monounsaturated fats – these include fibre-rich nuts, seeds and avocados – helps to lower levels of LDL and triglycerides in the blood, without lowering the healthy high-density lipoproteins (HDL), which carry cholesterol away from the tissues and back to the liver and decrease the risk of cardiovascular disease.

PROMOTING WEIGHT LOSS

Obesity is a growing risk to the health of people in developed nations. This is partly due to our modern lifestyles including our reliance on cars and desk-bound jobs. We eat more high-calorie foods that are dense in sugar and saturated fat, and we eat cheaper, faster foods, encouraged by the marketing of junk food and its convenience.

Weight control means maintaining a healthy weight that is right for your body. Balancing the amount of energy consumed with the amount used is essential to maintain this. If the food you eat provides more calories than you burn, your body will store the excess as fat. Ultimately, this could lead to obesity and associated health risks.

Losing weight should theoretically be a simple task, yet many of us find it incredibly difficult. Nearly two-thirds of the UK adult population is overweight and nearly half of these are in the obese category. The body mass index (BMI) is based on a ratio of your weight to your height and you can calculate yours using online websites such as the NHS. It is not used to diagnose obesity, however, because people who are very muscular can have a high BMI despite not having much fat, but it is a useful indication of whether you are a healthy weight. A healthy weight is defined as having a BMI of between 18.5 and 25. If your BMI is between 25 and 29.9, you are classified as overweight, and if your BMI is 30 or over, as obese, although BMI is not the only tool which is used to diagnose obesity.

Eating more fibre can help you to lose weight because it is filling and helps you to stay feeling full because the food stays in the stomach for longer while it is processed. Fibre-rich foods require more chewing, which can increase the secretion of a hormone in the gut that decreases appetite and plays a vital role in satiety.

A BALANCED DIET IS KEY

For healthy and sustained weight loss, you should eat a balanced and varied fibre-rich diet that reduces calories to a safe level without sacrificing essential nutrients. This will encourage long-term eating habits that you can continue to follow when you have reached a desirable weight. A fibre-rich diet is a great way to lose weight, but you should remember that fibre itself doesn't fuel your body or provide nutrients. Ultra-high fibre 'diet' products and 'weight-loss' supplements should be avoided, as they can reduce the amount of nutrients you absorb, especially minerals such as iron and calcium. If you embark on a restrictive long-term weight-loss diet, consider taking a mineral and vitamin supplement.

HOW MUCH FIBRE DO YOU NEED?

As mentioned earlier, current UK guidelines say that our intake of dietary fibre should increase to around 30g a day as part of a healthy balanced diet, yet most adults fall woefully short of this goal and are eating less than half this amount. This recommendation was made in 2015 and it is for optimum health. Before then, it was 18g per day and this should be the absolute minimum you should aim for.

There are many simple ways to introduce more fibre into our diet. A few decades ago, it was trendy to sprinkle wheat bran on everything from breakfast cereals to soups and casseroles. We now know that eating a large amount of pure wheat bran isn't good for you because it is high in phytates, which can interfere in the absorption of nutrients such as iron and calcium. It's important to obtain fibre from a wide variety of sources so that you get a good intake of both soluble and insoluble fibre, and you also benefit from the other many nutrients they contain.

When increasing fibre in your diet, make changes gradually and over a few weeks, rather than immediately increasing your intake from a low- to a high-fibre diet. This will allow the natural bacteria in your digestive system to adjust. Adding too much fibre too quickly might cause bloating and cramping, so take it slowly and make small changes in the first few days. Switching from white bread, pasta and rice to wholemeal or wholegrain alternatives for some of your meals is a good start.

The fibre and fluid connection

It's important to drink plenty of non-alcoholic fluids as part of a healthy diet, and in climates such as the UK you should aim to drink at least 1.2 litres (six 200ml glasses) a day to prevent dehydration, as mentioned previously. You will need more on very hot days and in warmer climates, or if you suffer from constipation. This doesn't have to be just water, but you should avoid too many caffeinated drinks such as coffee, tea and soft drinks containing caffeine, as these are diuretics (decaffeinated coffee and teas are fine).

Fibre absorbs fluid in the gut, so you'll need to drink more as your intake increases. Some foods, especially fruit and vegetables, have a high water content, which can offset the amount you need to drink; these include cucumber, melons, tomatoes, oranges and apples, which all have a water content of over 85 per cent.

FIBRE-RICH FOODS

There are five main groups of fibre-rich foods, and you should try to add some of each to your daily diet:

1 Grains such as wheat, oats, barley and rye – these are the main ingredients of wholegrain breakfast cereals including porridge, wholegrain and wholemeal breads, wholewheat pasta, wholegrain and brown rice
2 Pulses, such as chickpeas, red kidney beans and red and green lentils

3 Nuts and seeds
4 Fruit; fresh, dried, canned and frozen
5 Vegetables, including root vegetables and potatoes, and leafy greens and canned and frozen versions

WHOLESOME GRAINS

A whole grain is a grain that has not been overly processed or refined. It consists of the bran, germ and endosperm inside an inedible outer coating known as the hull, which is removed from the grain. The bran is the inner covering, which protects the seed, and is an excellent source of fibre. The germ is the potential new plant and is a great source of protein, vitamins and minerals. The endosperm is the source of carbohydrates, mostly starch. When grains are highly processed, the hull, bran and germ are all removed, to make a refined product such as white flour. Whole grains are not refined to this extent, so they retain all the beneficial nutrients and fibre.

HEALTHY PULSES

Low in fat, almost all pulses – dried beans, lentils and peas – contain a near-perfect balance of protein and starchy carbohydrate. Pulses are a useful source of protein for those who are trying to cut down on their meat and dairy intake, or who are vegetarian or vegan. Most pulses are excellent sources of both soluble and insoluble fibre.

NUTRITIOUS NUTS AND SEEDS

Nuts and seeds are nutritional superstars. A valuable source of protein, they are low in saturated fat and salt, and are cholesterol-free. Some nuts and seeds are rich in the healthy omega-3 fat, especially flax seeds (linseeds), chia seeds and walnuts. All are good sources of vitamins, particularly the B vitamins, as well as calcium. They are rich in soluble fibre.

FIVE-A-DAY FRUIT AND VEGETABLES

There is universal agreement among government nutritionists that we should all eat a minimum of five servings of fruit and vegetables each day, not counting potatoes. Many recommend that we should eat seven servings for optimum nutrition. The five-a-day campaign was introduced to raise public awareness, but a recent survey has found that fewer than one in five adults in the UK actually manage to consume this amount. It's a good idea to include a wide variety of fruit and vegetables in your diet, as different types contain different combinations of nutrients, including vitamins, minerals and antioxidants. Fresh, frozen, canned and dried fruit and vegetables can all be counted, and they don't have to be served separately. Vegetables such as onion, leek, and so on, in soups and casseroles count as a portion, too.

WHAT COUNTS AS A PORTION?

- 1 medium glass (125ml) of fruit or vegetable juice (this only counts as one portion per day, no matter how much you drink).
- 1 medium piece of fruit, such as an apple, pear, orange, nectarine or a slice of melon.
- 2 small fruits, such as satsumas, plums or kiwi fruit or 2 slices of mango.
- A large handful of small fruits such as grapes, cherries, blueberries or strawberries.
- 3 dried fruits such as apricots, prunes or figs (this only counts as one portion per day, no matter how many you eat).
- 6 tbsp canned fruit such as chopped peaches or pineapple chunks.
- ½ avocado, red, yellow or green pepper.
- 3 tbsp cooked vegetables such as mushrooms, peas, pak choi or sweetcorn.
- 3 tbsp cooked pulses such as red lentils, chickpeas or red kidney beans (this only counts as one portion per day no matter how much you eat).
- A cereal-sized bowl of salad such as lettuce leaves, watercress or raw spinach.

MEAL PLANNING

At first, increasing the amount of fibre in your diet to 30g might seem daunting, but planning your day's meals and snacks in advance will help you to work towards achieving this amount.

A sample menu idea:

BREAKFAST:
Overnight Oats (page 32) topped with 1 medium sliced banana: 2.5g fibre
or
1 slice of wholemeal toast with 1 tbsp Apricot Spread (page 36): 2.5g fibre

MID-MORNING SNACK:
3 Digestive Biscuits (page 184): 1.5g fibre

LUNCH:
Chicken Satay Wrap (page 60): 3.9g fibre
1 slice of Carrot and Coconut Cake (page 174): 3.3g fibre
or
A portion of Baked Vegetable Crisps (page 66): 3.3g fibre

AFTERNOON SNACK:
1 pear: 2.2g fibre
or
2 Cheese and Seed Oatcakes (page 186): 2.2g fibre

DINNER:
Lamb Tagine served with a crunchy salad (page 112): 8.5g fibre
Wholewheat Couscous (70g raw weight): 3.1g fibre
Chocolate and Avocado Mousse (page 156) 5g fibre

Total: 30g fibre

FIVE EASY WAYS TO BOOST YOUR FIBRE INTAKE

1 Eat more fruit and vegetables, at least five portions a day (see page 16).

2 Start the day with wholewheat breakfast cereal, which is naturally high in fibre, rather than adding neat wheat bran to your breakfast. Alternatively, try a bowl of porridge (some have added oat bran, which is great for lowering cholesterol), or make your own Granola (page 28). Now and then, top with fresh fruit such as berries, or sprinkle with seeds such as sunflower, pumpkin or flax seeds (linseeds). You can also use wholewheat breakfast cereals in baking, in coatings and for topping fruit crumbles.

3 Switch to wholegrain foods such as wholewheat pasta, brown rice and wholemeal bread rather than refined versions. Experiment with other grains such as barley, bulgar wheat, wholewheat couscous and quinoa. If you're not keen on wholemeal bread, try granary or rye breads, or compromise with versions that are part wholemeal, part white, or have high-fibre additions such as seeds or oats. There are lots of products with added fibre around, such as white pasta with oat fibre and cream crackers with added vegetable fibre.

4 Add a few cooked pulses such as red kidney beans or chickpeas to casseroles and stews; they add fibre and stretch the meat further. Even if you are not vegetarian, eat at least one meat-free main meal a week, based on pulses; they are high in protein and incredibly good for you.

5 Make snacks count: nuts and dried fruits are both high in fibre and nutrients (although they are high in calories, so don't have more than a handful if you are trying to lose weight). Low-fat popcorn and Baked Vegetable Crisps (see page 66) are also good snack choices.

FIBRE AND CHILDREN

Children under the age of sixteen don't need as much fibre as older teenagers and adults, but most still don't get nearly enough. The current recommendations are:

- 2 to 5-year-olds need about 15g fibre daily
- 5 to 11-year-olds need about 20g fibre daily
- 11 to 16-year-olds need about 25g fibre daily

It is important to introduce lots of different types of fruit and vegetables at an early age so that babies and toddlers get used to and enjoy a wide range of flavours and textures. The under twos can occasionally have wholegrain foods such as wholemeal pasta, rice and wholemeal bread, but not too often, as wholegrain foods can fill them up before they have taken in the calories and nutrients needed. After the age of two, you can gradually introduce a few more whole grains.

SMART SHOPPING

Food labels contain a wealth of information and can be useful when you are making healthier choices. They can help you decide not just which foods to buy but also while comparing different brands and varieties. Food labelling regulations produce standard definitions relating to the fibre content per portion size as well as per 100g. To carry the strap label 'source of fibre', the product must contain at least 3g fibre per serving. To be labelled 'high fibre', it must have at least 6g fibre per serving or at least 3g per 100 kcal.

FIBRE-RICH FOODS

The following charts show some of the best sources of fibre and some of the ingredients that you'll find included in the recipes in this book.

GRAINS
Brown rice 100g serving, boiled 0.8g
Bran flakes 1 bowl, 30g serving 3.9g
Flax seeds, whole or ground 1 tbsp 2.0g
Granary bread (1 medium slice) 1.5g
Oat bran 1 tbsp 1.0g
Oats 100g 7.0g
Porridge, cooked, 1 bowl, 200g serving 1.6g
Rye bread (1 medium slice) 1.1g
Wheatgerm 1 tbsp 1.0g
Wholemeal bread (1 medium slice) 2.1g
Wholewheat couscous, boiled 100g serving 2.7g
Wholemeal pitta bread (1 medium) 4.1g
Wholemeal spaghetti, boiled 100g serving 3.5g
Wholemeal tortilla wrap (1 medium 40g) 1.7g

PULSES AND LENTILS
Baked beans 100g serving 3.5g
Chickpeas, cooked 100g serving 4.1g
Kidney beans, cooked 100g serving 6.2g
Lentils (green), cooked 100g serving 3.8g
Lentils (red split), cooked 100g serving 1.9g

NUTS AND SEEDS
Almonds 100g 7.4g
Brazil nuts 100g 4.3g
Desiccated coconut 100g 13.7g
Hazelnuts 100g 6.5g
Peanuts 100g 6.2g
Peanut butter 1 tbsp 0.9g

Pumpkin seeds 100g 5.3g
Sesame seeds 100g 7.9g
Sunflower seeds 100g 6.0g
Walnuts 100g 3.5g

FRUIT
Apple (with skin) 1 medium 1.8g
Apricots (dried, ready-to-eat) 100g 6.3g
Banana 1 medium 1.1g
Dates (dried) 100g 3.4g
Figs (dried, ready-to-eat) 100g 6.9g
Kiwi fruit each 1.1g
Orange each 2.7g
Peach each 1.7g
Pear each 3.3g
Prunes (canned in juice) 100g serving 6g
Prunes (dried, ready-to-eat) 100g 5.7g
Raisins or sultanas 100g 2g
Raspberries 100g serving 2.5g

VEGETABLES
Avocado 1 medium 10.0g
Beansprouts, raw 100g serving 1.9g
Beetroot, cooked 100g serving 2.8g
Broccoli, cooked 100g serving 2.3g
Brussels sprouts, cooked 100g serving 3.1g
Carrots, cooked 100g serving 2.5g
Celery stick, 1 medium 0.6g
Peas, cooked 80g serving 4.1g
Potato, baked with skin 1 medium 2.6g
Sweet potato, cooked 100g serving 2.3g
Spring greens, cooked 100g serving 2.6g
Spring onion 1 medium 0.4g
Sweetcorn, canned 100g serving 2.3g
Tomatoes 1 medium whole fresh 1.5g
Tomatoes 400g can 4.0g

BASIC PREPARATION FOR YOUR STORE CUPBOARD

Many simple, fibre-rich ingredients are available in cans, packets or come frozen, and it's worth keeping a good stock of these. Others are cheaper and simple to prepare at home yourself when you have the time.

DATE SYRUP

Rich in minerals, especially calcium, potassium and magnesium, this syrupy sweetener can be used in many recipes instead of honey, golden syrup or maple syrup and is delicious drizzled over yogurt. It has a distinctive date flavour and a rich dark brown colour, so you need to consider this before using it in cooking, as it will dramatically alter the taste and colour of the finished dish.

Commercial date syrup is extracted from dates with the date pulp removed, which means that it has none of the health-promoting fibre. This homemade version is simple to make and contains whole dates.

MAKES ABOUT 300ML
100g pitted ready-to-eat dates, preferably Medjool
150ml boiling water
2 tsp lemon juice

1 Put the dates in a heatproof bowl and pour over the boiling water. Cover the bowl with a lid to retain the heat, then leave for 1 hour to cool and soften the dates.

2 Tip the mixture into a high-speed blender (you'll need a powerful one to get a completely smooth date syrup; otherwise, press the syrup through a fine plastic or stainless steel sieve to remove any larger lumps), add the lemon juice and blend until smooth. Store in glass jars or bottles in the fridge for up to 6 weeks.

BREADCRUMBS

It's not possible to buy wholemeal breadcrumbs, but they are quick and easy to make yourself, with the advantage that they are best made from bread which is two to three days old, so this is a great way to use up slightly stale or dry bread. Fresh breadcrumbs are soft in texture and absorbent, so they swell when mixed with liquid or slightly wet ingredients, where they often act as a binder. Dried breadcrumbs are finer and are used to crumb-coat foods, often before frying or oven baking, to give them a crisp and crunchy covering.

MAKES ABOUT 175G (depending on size and thickness of bread)
4 slices of day-old wholemeal bread, crusts removed, if you prefer

1   To make fresh breadcrumbs, tear the bread into pieces. Put into a food processor and whizz to make fine (or coarse, if you prefer) breadcrumbs.
2   To make dried breadcrumbs, tip the breadcrumbs onto a baking tray and allow them to dry out in a warm oven (after it's been used for cooking or switched to its lowest setting) for 10–15 minutes until dry, but not beginning to colour. Stir halfway through. Remove from the oven and allow to cool completely.
3   Use the breadcrumbs straight away or freeze if fresh; if dried, store in an airtight container for up to 4 weeks.

BEANS AND PULSES

You can purchase many types of pulses in 400g cans, but for those varieties you use a lot – in this book you'll find recipes that include chickpeas, black-eyed beans, black beans, flageolet beans, cannellini beans, borlotti beans and pinto beans – it's worth buying packets of dried beans, cooking them in bulk then freezing them in convenient-sized batches.

Soaking beans Pulses are dried so that they can be preserved for many months, keeping the protein and nutrient content. They need to be soaked to rehydrate them and to help them cook quicker. How long pulses need to be soaked depends on the variety as well as the length of time they have been stored.

Lentils and split peas don't need soaking, but most other beans and chickpeas should be soaked for at least 8 hours. As a general rule, soak until the beans have plumped up enough so that there is no wrinkling remaining on the skin. You can soak pulses for up to a day, but in warm weather or a heated kitchen you should put the bowl in the fridge if soaking for longer than 8 hours. After soaking, drain the pulses and rinse.

Cooking beans After rinsing, cook the soaked beans in fresh water. There are toxic proteins contained in the outer layers of most pulses, which cannot be digested and can make you unwell (red kidney beans are particularly high in these). These are destroyed with a short period of rapid boiling, so it's recommended to do a rapid boil for the first 10 minutes of cooking time for most pulses (this isn't necessary with chickpeas, split peas or lentils). You can then reduce the heat to a gentle simmer for the remaining cooking time.

Once the pulses are gently simmering, skim the froth from the surface, then partly cover the pan and leave them to cook gently until the pulses are tender, topping up with more boiling water, if needed. Do not add salt to the cooking water, because this will toughen the pulses and prolong the cooking time.

You should also avoid adding bicarbonate of soda. This is sometimes recommended in old cookery books as it shortens the cooking time, but it also affects the flavour and destroys some of the nutrients. The length of the simmering time depends on the variety of pulse and how dry it is; for example, pinto beans can take 45 minutes to 1½ hours. Check the packet for a guide to the pulse you are cooking, but also check the pulses are cooked; they should be completely tender but not mushy or beginning to break up. Although you might be cooking them for a little longer in your chosen recipe, if the sauce contains an acidic ingredient such as tomatoes or vinegar, the pulses will not become any softer. After cooking, drain well and leave to cool, then pack into re-usable freezer containers or plastic bags, freeze and label. The drained weight of a 400g tin of pulses is about 250g, so this is a good amount to divide your cooked beans into. Cooked beans can be frozen for up to 4 months.

Breakfasts and Brunches

Try to make time for breakfast; it's a great way to start clocking up your fibre and five-a-day intake. It's easy to start the day with a bowl of wholegrain cereal or a couple of slices of wholemeal toast and a fibre-rich topping such as Apricot Spread (page 36) or peanut butter. Breakfast normally follows a period of fasting as you sleep, so it's important to refuel for the day ahead, if you want to avoid a mid-morning energy dip.

Oats are a particularly nutritious choice as they provide soluble fibre, which can help lower 'bad' LDL cholesterol. You'll find several ways to use them here, including Crunchy Granola Cereal (page 28) and Overnight Oats (page 32). If you decide to start the day with a bowl of cereal, squeeze in more fibre by topping with some fresh fruit, a few raisins or some chopped dried apricots, and add a sprinkling of ground flax (linseed), or other seeds or nuts.

When you have more time, perhaps a brunch at weekends, there are plenty of other options here, such as Buttermilk Banana Pancakes (page 34) and Oat Bran and Honey Muffins (page 40); get the ingredients together the night before, so that they take only minutes in the morning to prepare. Occasionally though, you might be running late and simply not have time to sit and eat. On those days, it's good to have some Breakfast Bars (page 42) in the fridge or freezer, individually wrapped and ready-to-go.

Finally, eating a healthy fibre-rich breakfast doesn't mean that you have to forgo a traditional full English, if this is a dish you enjoy now and then; poach the eggs instead of frying them and grill the bacon on a rack until crisp to reduce the fat content, adding some halved tomatoes and mushrooms to the grill pan. Serve with a slice of wholemeal toast and add a generous helping of baked beans to your plate to up the fibre content even more.

Crunchy Granola Cereal

Shop-bought granola and crunchy breakfast cereals can be high in fat and sugar. This version still contains both, but considerably less than most commercial varieties. Making your own allows you to tailor the mixture to your liking so that you can enjoy your favourite fruit and nut combination.

SERVES 8

250g porridge (rolled) oats
3 tbsp sesame seeds
50g chopped hazelnuts
50g desiccated coconut
100ml rapeseed oil
4 tbsp clear honey
1 tbsp light brown sugar
1 tsp finely grated orange zest (optional)
100g dried fruit, such as sultanas, chopped dried apricots or cranberries
dairy or non-dairy milk or yogurt, to serve

1 Preheat the oven to 180°C/fan oven 160°C/gas 4. Put the oats, sesame seeds, hazelnuts and coconut in a bowl and mix together.

2 Put 150ml water into a jug and add the oil, honey, sugar and orange zest, if using. Whisk together. Drizzle over the dry ingredients (stop and whisk the liquid again occasionally to keep it well blended), then mix everything together thoroughly.

3 Spread the mixture out on a large non-stick baking tray. Bake for 20–25 minutes, turning the clumps of granola twice during cooking, so that they brown evenly. The mixture should be a light golden brown and completely dry; if not, cook for a further 5 minutes.

4 Remove from the oven and allow the mixture to cool completely. Mix in the dried fruit and store in an airtight container. Serve with milk or yogurt.

FOR EXTRA FIBRE

Scatter a handful of sunflower seeds over the mixture 5 minutes before the end of the cooking time, so that they are lightly toasted. You could also add 2–3 tbsp oat bran, wheatgerm or ground flax seeds to the granola when stirring in the dried fruit. If you like, top your bowl of cereal with some fresh fruit as well, such as sliced bananas, chopped tinned peaches or fresh berries.

NUTRITIONAL NOTE

Rapeseed oil is ideal for this recipe as it has a nutty flavour and a distinctive rich golden colour that complements the granola. Containing omegas-3, 6 and 9, it is high in beneficial mono-unsaturated fats and is one of the only unblended oils that can be heated to a high temperature without spoiling its antioxidant properties.

Suitable for vegetarians. For vegans, use agave syrup instead of honey.

Quinoa Berry Porridge

Here, a mixture of highly nutritious quinoa flakes are used together with traditional porridge oats to give this breakfast a lovely creamy finish. Frozen berries are much cheaper when fresh ones aren't in season and are a great freezer stand-by.

SERVES 4

600ml milk (skimmed, semi-skimmed or non-dairy such as almond milk), plus extra if needed

a small pinch of salt (optional)

100g quinoa flakes

50g porridge (rolled) oats

100g frozen mixed berries, such as blueberries, raspberries, cherries

honey, maple syrup, agave syrup or soft brown sugar, to serve (optional)

1   Pour the milk into a heavy-based saucepan, add the salt, if using, then sprinkle over the quinoa flakes. Slowly bring to the boil and simmer for 5 minutes, stirring occasionally.

2   Add the porridge oats and stir well. Bring the mixture back to the boil and simmer for 3 minutes, stirring frequently.

3   Add the frozen fruit, bring back to simmering point and cook for a further 1–2 minutes until the porridge is thick and creamy and the fruit is warmed through. Stir carefully and not too often at this stage to keep the berries whole.

4   Turn off the heat and stir in a splash of extra milk if you prefer your porridge a little thinner. Spoon into bowls and serve immediately with a drizzle of honey if you like.

FOR EXTRA FIBRE

Stir a spoonful or two of toasted seeds, wheatgerm or oat bran into the porridge before serving. You could also sprinkle over a few toasted flaked almonds, if you like. You can buy many types of nuts, such as hazelnuts and flaked almonds, ready toasted. To toast yourself, put on a baking tray in a single layer and bake in a low oven (150°C/fan oven 130°C/gas 2) for 10-12 minutes until golden. You can also toast them in a dry frying pan over a low heat, stirring frequently to make sure that they colour evenly. Watch carefully, as they can burn quickly.

NUTRITIONAL NOTE

Quinoa is a high-fibre food with both soluble (a third) and insoluble (two-thirds) fibre. High in protein, it contains all nine essential amino acids (the protein building blocks) as well as B-vitamins and minerals including calcium and iron. Quinoa flakes are quinoa seeds that have been rolled flat in a similar process to the way porridge oats are made. They have a slightly firmer texture than oats when made into porridge and take a little longer to cook.

Suitable for vegetarians. Vegans should use a non-dairy milk and serve the porridge with maple or agave syrup or soft brown sugar.

Overnight Oats

A bowl of steaming hot porridge is a welcoming start on a wintry morning, but in the heat of summer you can still enjoy the benefits of oats with this Bircher-style breakfast which can be prepared the night before for a relaxed start to the day.

SERVES 6

125g porridge (rolled) oats

50g unsalted nuts such as almonds, or mixed nuts, roughly chopped

1 tbsp ground flax seeds (linseeds)

¼ tsp ground cinnamon

1 large eating apple

4 tbsp apple or orange juice

300ml natural yogurt

honey, maple syrup or date syrup (page 23) for drizzling (optional)

1   Put the oats, nuts, flax and cinnamon in a bowl and mix together. Leaving the peel on the apple, quarter, core and coarsely grate it into a small bowl, then immediately sprinkle over the apple or orange juice and stir to coat – this will help to stop it from going brown.

3   Add the grated apple and yogurt to the dry ingredients and stir together. Leave the mixture in the bowl and cover with cling film, or divide it among six small glass pots with lids or suitable small containers. Chill in the fridge overnight; the mixture will thicken as the oats soak up the moisture. Serve with a drizzle of honey, if you like.

Alternative toppings (each serves 2)

Strawberry and blueberry Purée 75g hulled fresh or defrosted frozen strawberries and 2 tsp honey or maple syrup (optional) until smooth. Use to top the oats and scatter with fresh blueberries.

Mango and coconut Purée 100g fresh mango with 2 tbsp orange juice or pineapple juice. Use to top the oats and scatter with coconut flakes.

Banana and chocolate Mix 4 tbsp yogurt with 1 tbsp cocoa or cacao powder and 1 tbsp date syrup (see page 23). Use to top the oats and add sliced banana and a sprinkling of chopped 70 per cent (or more) dark chocolate.

TIP

Use a mild-tasting creamy bio yogurt for the best flavour and to reduce the desire to sweeten this breakfast. Once made, the overnight oats will keep in the fridge for up to 3 days.

VARIATIONS

If you like, reduce the amount of oats to 100g and add 1 tbsp chia seeds to the overnight oat mixture. You could also use some quinoa flakes (substitute an equal weight) instead of some of the oats for a protein boost.

Suitable for vegetarians. Vegans should use a non-dairy yogurt such as soya and serve with maple or date syrup.

Buttermilk Banana Pancakes

Although the name suggests otherwise, buttermilk is low in fat and gives these wholemeal mini pancakes a lovely light texture. Serve them hot straight from the pan to enjoy them at their best. For extra fibre, drizzle them with a little date syrup (see page 23).

SERVES 4 (MAKES 12 PANCAKES)
175g wholemeal self-raising flour
50g white self-raising flour
a pinch of salt
25g caster sugar
2 eggs, separated
300ml buttermilk
1 large banana, thinly sliced
sunflower or coconut oil, for frying
date syrup (page 23) or honey or maple syrup (optional), to
   serve

1   Sift the flours and salt into a large bowl, adding the bran left in the sieve. Stir in the sugar, then make a well in the centre. Add the egg yolks, buttermilk and 1 tablespoon of cold water, and gradually work in the flour mixture using a wooden spoon to make a smooth, thick batter.

2   Whisk the egg whites in a clean bowl until stiff, then gently fold into the batter with a large metal spoon. Fold in the banana slices.

3   Heat a griddle or a large non-stick frying pan over a medium-high heat, then lightly grease with a teaspoon of oil. Add large spoonfuls of the batter to the hot pan to make 3 or 4 pancakes at a time, spacing them apart.

4   Cook for 2–3 minutes until golden and firm, and bubbles appear on the surface of the pancakes. Turn them over and cook for a further 1–2 minutes until the underside is golden.

5 Remove from the pan and serve straight away or keep warm while cooking the remaining pancakes, lightly greasing the pan between each batch. Serve the pancakes drizzled with date syrup, if you like.

TIP

Traditionally, buttermilk was the liquid left after the creamy part of the milk had been churned into butter, although commercial buttermilk is now usually made by adding a culture to skimmed milk to sour and thicken it. For an easy substitute, add a teaspoon of lemon juice to 300ml skimmed or semi-skimmed milk and leave to stand at room temperature for about 15 minutes before using.

FOR EXTRA FIBRE

Add a few sultanas, raisins or other chopped dried fruit such as apricots to the mixture with the sliced banana.

Suitable for vegetarians.

Apricot Spread

Bought jams, conserves and spreads often have a low fruit content and a high amount of sugar and additives. This fruity jam uses dried fruit, so it can be made at any time of the year. Dried apricots are rich in fibre and a good source of iron.

MAKES ABOUT 400G
250g dried apricots
1 tsp vanilla extract

1 Snip the apricots into quarters using kitchen scissors. Put them in a heavy-based saucepan, pour over about 300ml water, cover the pan with a lid and leave to soak for 30 minutes.
2 Check the water level and pour in a little more if needed to make sure the apricots are just covered. Slowly bring to the boil, then cover the pan and simmer gently for 20–25 minutes until the apricots are very soft and pulpy. Check the mixture frequently towards the end of the cooking time, stirring so that they don't stick to the base. If necessary, add a little more water to the pan.
3 Turn off the heat and allow the mixture to stand for 10 minutes, still covered with the lid. Remove the lid and leave until tepid.
4 Spoon the apricot mixture into a food processor or blender, add the vanilla, then blend for just a few seconds to make a slightly chunky spread.
5 Spoon the apricot spread into a clean jar or jars and leave to cool completely. Put on the lids and keep in the fridge for up to 3 weeks.

TIPS

- If you prefer not to use a food processor, snip the apricots into smaller pieces before soaking.
- As well as a delicious spread for crusty bread and toast, this is also good served on top of porridge, rice pudding and sponge puddings.

VARIATIONS

- For a fruitier-flavoured spread, make this using apple, orange or pineapple juice instead of all or part of the water.
- This spread can also be made with dried peaches instead of apricots and flavoured with rose water or orange flower water instead of vanilla extract.

NUTRITIONAL NOTE

As well as a high soluble-fibre content, dried apricots are naturally high in antioxidants, which help to guard against environmental damage from sunlight and pollution. They also provide good amounts of potassium and are a source of vitamin A and calcium.

Suitable for vegetarians and vegans.

Dried Fruit Compote

This delicious, fruity breakfast is made with dried fruit, so it can be enjoyed all year round. It's best made a day or two before serving to allow the flavours to develop and mingle. It can be served chilled or reheated and served warm on chilly days.

SERVES 4

600ml boiling water
1 Earl Grey teabag
1 vanilla pod
3 tbsp clear honey
500g good-quality ready-to-eat dried fruit, such as prunes, figs, apricots, pears, apple rings and cranberries
Greek yogurt or kefir yogurt, to serve

1   Pour the water into a heatproof jug, add the teabag and vanilla pod and leave to infuse for 5 minutes. Remove the teabag and discard. Stir the honey into the tea.
2   Put the fruit into a bowl and pour over the warm weak tea mixture, tucking the vanilla pod under the fruit. Leave until completely cool. Remove the vanilla pod.
3   Cover the bowl with cling film and put in the fridge. Leave the fruit to soak and soften for at least 12 hours before serving; most of the liquid will be absorbed.
4   Ladle the compote into bowls and serve chilled or at room temperature with yogurt. Alternatively, gently re-heat, either in the bowl in the microwave, or in a saucepan on the hob.

VARIATIONS

- For a spicier version, use 2 lemon and ginger teabags instead of the Earl Grey teabag and add a 2cm piece of peeled fresh root ginger or ½ cinnamon stick instead of the vanilla pod. You could also add a pared piece of lemon or orange zest when steeping the tea.
- Alternatively, use 2 fruit-flavoured teabags such as cranberry, strawberry or raspberry and add some dried fruit such as sour cherries or blueberries to the mix.
- You can also use fruit juice in the compote: steep the teabag in 300ml boiling water and when the mixture is cool, add 300ml clear apple or cranberry juice.

TIP

There's no need to discard the vanilla pod. Rinse it thoroughly under cold running water and leave it to dry. Keep for another recipe.

Suitable for vegetarians. Vegans should use agave syrup instead of honey and serve with a non-dairy yogurt such as soya.

Oat Bran and Honey Muffins

These lightly spiced muffins are perfect for a weekend brunch. To save time, measure out the dry and wet ingredients the night before – keep the wet mixture in the fridge overnight – ready to quickly mix and bake in the morning. These are also an excellent addition to lunchboxes.

MAKES 12

175g self-raising white flour
175g self-raising wholemeal flour
1 tsp ground cinnamon
½ tsp ground mixed spice
1 tsp baking powder
a pinch of salt
50g oat bran
5 tbsp soft light brown sugar
6 tbsp rapeseed or sunflower oil
3 tbsp clear honey
2 eggs, lightly beaten
250ml milk
100g sultanas
oil, for greasing (optional)

1 Sift the flours, cinnamon, spice, baking powder and salt into a mixing bowl, adding the bran left in the sieve. Stir in the oat bran and sugar. If keeping for the next day, cover with a clean tea towel.
2 In a separate bowl or jug, mix the oil, honey, eggs and milk together. Add the sultanas. If keeping for the next day, cover with cling film and store in the fridge.

3   Preheat the oven to 200°C/fan oven 180°C/gas 6. Remove the bowl or jug of wet ingredients from the fridge if you have chilled it overnight, and give the mixture a stir. Leave at room temperature for a few minutes while the oven is heating. Grease a 12-cup muffin tin or line the cups with paper muffin cases.
4   Make a hollow in the centre of the dry ingredients and pour in the wet ingredients. Mix briefly with a large metal spoon until just combined; stop mixing while the batter is still lumpy.
5   Spoon the batter into the prepared muffin cups or paper cases, dividing it evenly. Bake for 18–20 minutes until the tops are lightly browned and springy to the touch. Take care not to over-bake or the muffins might be dry. Cool in the tin for 5 minutes, then carefully remove the muffins and put on a wire rack. Serve warm or cold.

TIP

Muffins are best eaten on the same day of making, or frozen as soon as they are cool.

VARIATION

For blueberry muffins, leave out the sultanas and stir in 100g fresh or partially defrosted frozen blueberries when adding the wet ingredients to the dry. Reduce the milk to 225ml as the blueberries will add more moisture to the mix.

Suitable for vegetarians.

Breakfast Bars

These high-energy bars are perfect for days when you are too rushed for a sit-down breakfast and want something to eat on the go. Packed with oats, dried fruit, nuts and seeds, they also make a perfect snack or lunchbox treat.

MAKES 12-14
150g butter, plus extra for greasing
250g porridge (rolled) oats
100g dried apricots, finely chopped
50g raisins
50g unsalted peanuts, roughly chopped
50g ground almonds
50g sesame seeds
150g clear honey
200g demerara sugar

1　Preheat the oven to 190°C/fan oven 170°C/gas 5. Grease and line the base of a 23cm square tin with baking paper. Put the oats, apricots, raisins, peanuts, almonds and sesame seeds in a large bowl and mix together.
2　Put the butter, honey and sugar in a heavy-based saucepan and gently heat, stirring occasionally until the sugar has completely dissolved. Bring the mixture to the boil, then reduce the heat and gently simmer for 4 minutes. Pour over the dry ingredients and stir everything together.
3　Spoon and scrape the mixture into the prepared tin and bake for 20 minutes or until it turns a slightly darker golden-brown colour.
4　Remove from the oven and put the tin on a wire rack to cool completely, then chill in the fridge for an hour. Turn out and cut into 12 or 14 bars.

- You can vary the fruit and nut content of these bars to suit your own personal taste. Dried fruits such as cranberries, mango and pineapple all work well, as do different nuts such as walnuts or pecan nuts. Substitute whatever you like, but just make sure that the weights of ingredients remain the same.
- To resist the temptation of eating these all in one go (they are packed with nutrients and fibre but do have a fairly high fat and sugar content), wrap them individually in foil and store in the freezer ready to be removed when needed. You can add them to lunchboxes while they are still frozen; they will be defrosted by midday and will help to keep the contents of the lunchbox cool.

Suitable for vegetarians. Vegans should substitute a vegan baking margarine for the butter and agave syrup or coconut nectar syrup for the honey.

Pear and Raspberry Smoothie

Eating more fresh fruit is a simple way to increase your daily fibre intake, but don't forget that frozen and tinned fruit are useful too, especially when the fruit bowl is empty. This quick and easy shake is a great breakfast in a glass, especially for those who don't fancy eating much in the morning.

SERVES 2
300ml skimmed or semi-skimmed milk
4–5 tbsp Greek-style yogurt, to taste
125g drained tinned pears (from a tin of pears in juice)
75g frozen raspberries (no need to defrost first)
1 tbsp wheatgerm

1 Put all the ingredients in a blender or food processor and blend for 1–2 minutes until completely smooth and creamy.
2 Pour into 2 tall glasses and serve the smoothies straight away, while still thick and frothy.

TIPS

- A 400g can of pears will yield about 250g pears when drained. Keep the remaining juice to serve as a drink (delicious mixed with some apple juice) and the remaining pears to make a smoothie another day, or to enjoy as a snack or dessert.
- The frozen raspberries will make the smoothie icy cold; if you prefer, defrost the raspberries overnight in the fridge so that the drink is just slightly chilled. You can of course use fresh raspberries for this recipe.

FOR EXTRA FIBRE

Add a few dried apricots to the smoothie (soak them in the pear juice in the fridge overnight so that they are really soft) and add 2 tbsp porridge (rolled) oats.

NUTRITIONAL NOTE

As well as adding fibre, wheatgerm contains vitamin E and B vitamins and is great for adding to smoothies and sprinkling over breakfast cereals.

Suitable for vegetarians. Vegans should substitute a non-dairy milk – almond or hazelnut milk work well here – and use a non-dairy yogurt instead of Greek yogurt.

Lower-Fat Eggs Benedict

There are conflicting stories about the origins of this famous dish, but it was definitely created in New York in the 1920s. Traditionally served on English white muffins with bacon and a buttery hollandaise, here toasted wholemeal muffins, lean ham and a lower-fat yogurt hollandaise are used.

SERVES 4

1 tsp vinegar
4 medium or large eggs
4 wholemeal English muffins, halved
4 slices lean ham, about 50g in total

For the yogurt hollandaise:
1 tsp Dijon mustard
2 medium egg yolks
150ml full-fat Greek yogurt
salt and ground white pepper

1 To make the hollandaise, whisk the mustard and egg yolks together in a heatproof bowl and add the yogurt. Put the bowl over a pan of barely simmering water and cook for 12–14 minutes, stirring constantly until thick (the sauce will become thinner at first, but will then thicken). Remove from the heat and leave the bowl over the hot water to keep it warm.

2 Half-fill a frying pan with boiling water and stir in the vinegar. Put over a low heat so that the water is just simmering, then carefully break the eggs into the water, one at a time. Poach for 3–4 minutes, spooning the hot water over the eggs towards the end of cooking time, until the eggs are cooked to your liking.

3   Meanwhile, toast the muffins. Place one half of each on 4
    warmed plates (make sure the plates aren't too hot or the
    sauce will split when served). Top each muffin half with a
    slice of ham.
4   Remove the eggs from the pan using a slotted spoon. Briefly
    drain on kitchen paper to blot up excess water (trim off any
    ragged edges of egg white with kitchen scissors, if you like),
    then place a poached egg on top of each slice of ham.
5   Season the yogurt hollandaise with salt and pepper and
    spoon over the eggs. Serve immediately with the remaining
    toasted muffin halves.

TIP

Use full-fat Greek yogurt for this recipe, rather than half-fat or
Greek-style yogurt which might separate on heating.

FOR EXTRA FIBRE

Serve the eggs Benedict with grilled tomatoes and mushrooms or
maybe a few steamed asparagus spears.

Soups, Salads and Snacks

This chapter offers dishes for all sorts of occasions, from light lunches and simple supper dishes to shareable platters, which are great for casual entertaining. If you are choosing recipes from this chapter to serve for lunch, they should be sustaining enough to keep your energy levels up throughout the day without being too heavy. It's a good idea to plan what you are going to eat in the evening as well, so that you get a different range of fibre-rich foods.

Easy to prepare, soups retain all the nutrients in their cooking liquid. Vegetables play a vital role, either as the main ingredient, as in my Green Pea and Flageolet Bean Soup (page 52) and Roasted Red Pepper and Tomato Soup (page 58), or by bringing taste, texture and colour to lentils or tender chicken, as in the Chunky Vegetable and Lentil Soup (page 50) and Chicken Noodle Soup (page 54).

Salads packed with vitamin-rich fruit and vegetables, usually raw but sometimes lightly cooked, are a great way to hit your fibre target. Boosted with protein, they can make well-balanced meals that really satisfy. For those days when you fancy a salad but are looking for something more substantial, grains such as barley and wholewheat couscous help boost your intake of both healthy complex carbohydrates and fibre, so they are great ingredients to keep in your store cupboard.

Few of us just stick to three meals a day, and snacks have become an increasingly important part of our diet. If you snack, try to eat them mid-morning and mid-afternoon to prevent energy dips and make sure that they count towards your fibre goal. Try some Lower-Fat Hummus (page 64) with a few Cheese and Seed Oatcakes (page 186) or share a bowl of Baked Vegetable Crisps and Tortilla Chips (page 66).

Chunky Vegetable and Lentil Soup

This warming, lightly spiced soup is robust and satisfying – perfect on a chilly day. Red lentils thicken the soup and are a good inexpensive source of protein. Serve with some crusty wholemeal toast or rolls for extra fibre.

SERVES 4

150g red split lentils
1 tbsp rapeseed or olive oil
1 onion, chopped
1 tsp hot chilli powder or a large pinch of dried chilli flakes
2 carrots, diced
1 celery stick, halved lengthways and chopped
1 sweet potato, diced
1 litre vegetable stock
2 leaves green cabbage, such as Savoy, or spring greens, thick
    central stalks removed, leaves finely shredded
salt and freshly ground black pepper
hot wholemeal toast or rolls, to serve

1 Put the lentils in a small bowl and pour over plenty of cold water to cover them. Leave to soak for a few minutes while cooking the vegetables.
2 Heat the oil in a large non-stick saucepan over a medium heat, add the onion and gently fry for 5 minutes or until soft but not coloured. Stir in the chilli powder, carrots, celery and sweet potato.
3 Drain the lentils thoroughly in a sieve and add to the pan with 900ml of the stock. Bring to the boil, then half-cover the pan with a lid and simmer over a low heat for 10 minutes.
4 Add the cabbage, re-cover the pan and simmer for a further 8–10 minutes until all the vegetables are tender. Add the remaining stock if you like your soup a little thinner. Season to taste with salt and pepper. Ladle the soup into warmed bowls and serve straight away with hot wholemeal toast.

TIPS

- You can use any combination of root vegetables in this soup, such as parsnips, swede or a small amount of potato, and include squash as well, if you like, such as pumpkin or butternut squash (but add a little less stock if using these, as they have a high water content). Keep the total weight of vegetables roughly the same.
- If you prefer your soup a little thicker, ladle a third of the soup into a blender, allow it to cool a little, then blend until smooth. Tip the purée back into the pan and gently re-heat the soup until piping hot.

Suitable for vegetarians and vegans.

Green Pea and Flageolet Bean Soup with Minted Yogurt

Flageolet beans are a pale green colour with a delicate yet distinctive taste. Here they are combined with peas to make an attractive soup, finished with a swirl of creamy Greek-style yogurt and fresh mint.

SERVES 4
1 tbsp olive oil
2 leeks, thinly sliced
1 celery stick, thinly sliced
1 medium potato, about 150g
1 litre boiling vegetable stock
200g fresh or frozen peas
400g can flageolet beans, drained and rinsed
salt and freshly ground black pepper

For the minted yogurt:
6 tbsp Greek-style yogurt
2 tbsp chopped fresh mint

1   Heat the oil in a large heavy-based saucepan. Add the leeks and celery, and cook over a low heat for 5 minutes or until softened, stirring occasionally. Stir in the potato and cook for 3 minutes. Add the stock and bring to the boil. Half-cover the pan with a lid, reduce the heat and simmer gently for 10 minutes.
2   Stir in the peas and beans and season to taste with salt and pepper. Bring back to a gentle simmer and cook for a further 10 minutes. Turn off the heat and let the soup cool a little.
3   Purée the soup in a blender or food processor until smooth. Tip back into the pan and gently re-heat until piping hot.

4 Meanwhile, to make the minted yogurt, put the yogurt and mint in a small bowl and season with salt and pepper to taste. Stir together.

5 Ladle the soup into warmed bowls and serve each topped with a large spoonful of minted yogurt. Swirl into the soup and serve straight away.

FOR EXTRA FIBRE

Serve the soup with bagel 'crisps': slice wholemeal bagels vertically (from top to bottom) into thin rounds. Brush the cut sides with a little olive oil and sprinkle with a few sesame seeds if you like, then arrange on a baking tray and bake at 150°C/fan oven 130°C/gas 2 for about ten minutes until lightly toasted and crisp. Keep a close eye on them, as they burn easily. Serve with the soup.

NUTRITIONAL NOTE

Peas are high in both protein and fibre, and contain around 5.6g per 100g of each. They are also a good vegan source of iron, phosphorus (needed along with calcium for bone-building) and B vitamins.

Suitable for vegetarians. Vegans should use a non-dairy yogurt such as soya yogurt.

Chicken Noodle Soup

This is a simple, tasty meal-in-a-bowl soup with wholewheat noodles, which soak up the flavours and thicken the soup. Tender chicken pieces are complemented by diced carrots, celery, peas and sweetcorn, and a little milk stirred in at the end of cooking gives it a creamy finish.

SERVES 4

1 tbsp rapeseed or sunflower oil
1 small onion, finely chopped
1 celery stick, chopped
1 carrot, chopped
750ml boiling good-quality chicken stock
1 bay leaf
1 skinless chicken breast, about 175g
75g wholewheat egg noodles
200g can sweetcorn, drained
50g frozen peas, defrosted
100ml semi-skimmed milk
salt and freshly ground black pepper
wholemeal toast, to serve (optional)

1 Heat the oil in a heavy-based saucepan, add the onion and cook over a low heat for 5 minutes, stirring frequently. Add the celery and carrot and cook for a further 2 minutes, stirring.

2 Pour in the stock, add the bay leaf and bring to the boil. Reduce the heat, half-cover the pan with a lid and simmer for 4–5 minutes, while preparing the chicken.

3 Trim the chicken breast, if necessary, and cut into 1cm chunks. Add to the pan and simmer gently for 3 minutes. Break the noodles into smaller manageable pieces and add to the pan with the sweetcorn and peas. Simmer for 2–3 minutes or according to the instructions on the noodles, until the chicken, vegetables and noodles are all cooked and tender.

4   Turn off the heat and, when the soup stops simmering, stir in the milk and season with salt and pepper. Re-heat until the soup is steaming hot, but not boiling.

5   Remove and discard the bay leaf. Ladle the soup into warmed bowls and serve straight away with some wholemeal toast, if you like.

Variation

For a vegan version use a 200g packet of firm tofu, cut into 1cm cubes, instead of the chicken, adding it to the pan, then adding the noodles (make sure you select an egg-free brand), as soon as the stock comes back to the boil. Use vegetable stock instead of chicken stock and replace the dairy milk with a non-dairy milk such as almond milk (stir a little of the hot soup into the milk before adding it to the pan, as non-dairy milks are prone to separating if boiled).

Classic Minestrone

This substantial soup is packed with vegetables, beans and wholewheat pasta – the perfect choice for a simple meal on a cold day. It is a great recipe for a cook-ahead meal as the flavours mature and improve if it is chilled overnight then reheated for serving, so it's worth making double the quantity.

SERVES 4-6

1 tbsp olive oil

1 onion, finely chopped

1 garlic clove, finely chopped

150g dried cannellini or borlotti beans, soaked overnight and drained

1.5 litres unsalted vegetable stock or water

400g can chopped tomatoes

1 tbsp tomato purée

1 carrot, finely diced

150g celeriac, finely diced

150g pumpkin, butternut squash or swede, finely diced

1 bay leaf

150g potatoes, finely diced

100g green beans, cut into 2cm lengths

75g small wholewheat pasta shapes such as conchigliette (shells) or farfallini (bows)

100g green cabbage leaves, such as Savoy, very finely shredded

salt and freshly ground black pepper

Parmesan cheese, to serve

1 Heat the oil in a large heavy-based saucepan over a medium heat. Add the onion and cook for 5 minutes or until softened. Add the garlic and cook for a further minute, stirring, then add the beans and stock. Bring to a rapid boil and boil for 10 minutes, then reduce the heat, cover the pan and simmer for 30 minutes.

2 Add the tomatoes and tomato purée, carrot, celeriac, pumpkin and bay leaf. Bring back to simmering point and simmer for 10 minutes.

3 Stir in the potatoes and green beans, and simmer for a further 5 minutes. Stir in the pasta and cabbage and cook for a final 10 minutes or until the cannellini or borlotti beans, vegetables and pasta are all tender.

4 Turn off the heat and leave to stand for 2–3 minutes, then taste and season with salt and pepper. Ladle into warmed bowls and serve straight away with shavings of grated Parmesan cheese.

TIP

If you can't get any small wholewheat pasta shapes, break wholewheat spaghetti into short lengths and use those instead.

Suitable for vegetarians. Vegans should serve with a Parmesan-style vegan cheese.

Roasted Red Pepper and Tomato Soup

Roasting peppers intensifies their flavour and gives them a slightly smoky taste. This soup is fantastic served with crisp slices of pesto bread, which can be cooked in the oven at the same time as the peppers.

SERVES 4

3 large red peppers
1 brown or multi-grain baguette, about 30cm long
3 tbsp pesto
1 tbsp olive oil
1 onion, roughly chopped
1 garlic clove, crushed
300ml tomato passata
300ml boiling vegetable stock
4 tbsp crème fraîche
salt and freshly ground black pepper

1   Preheat the oven to 200°C/fan oven 180°C/gas 6. Line a large baking sheet with baking paper. Cut each pepper in half through the stalk, then remove the white membrane and seeds. Put on the baking sheet cut-side down and roast for 25–30 minutes until the skin is blistered and shrivelled. Leave on the baking sheet until cool enough to handle.

2   Meanwhile, make the pesto bread. Cut the baguette into 3.5cm thick slices, leaving the slices attached at the base. Holding the slices apart, spread each one thinly with pesto, then press back together. Wrap in foil and put on a baking sheet on an oven shelf below the peppers. Bake for 15 minutes or until the crust is crisp and slightly darker in colour.

3 While the peppers and bread are cooking, heat the oil in a large heavy-based saucepan. Add the onion and cook over a medium-low heat for 5–7 minutes until softened. Add the garlic and cook for a further 1 minute, stirring constantly. Turn off the heat and leave to cool.

4 Carefully peel the blistered skins off the peppers and discard. Roughly chop the peppers and put them into a blender or food processor. Add the cooked onion mixture and about two-thirds of the passata. Blend to a smooth purée.

5 Pour the puréed mixture back into the pan and add the remaining passata and stock. Season with salt and pepper. Heat the soup until piping hot, but do not boil. Ladle into warmed bowls and add a spoonful of crème fraîche to each. Serve straight away with slices of warm pesto bread.

TIP

You can also use orange or yellow peppers for this soup, but don't use green ones as they can have a slightly bitter flavour when roasted.

FOR EXTRA FIBRE

Add a celery stick and a carrot, both finely chopped, when cooking the onion. If they start to stick to the base of the pan, add a spoonful or two of the stock and cover with a pan lid for a few seconds, then stir and continue to cook.

Suitable for vegetarians. Vegans should omit the crème fraîche.

Chicken Satay Wraps

Peanut butter is a great source of fibre. Here it's used in a classic Indonesian satay sauce, which is drizzled over tender chunks of marinated chicken. Served in wholewheat tortillas for easy eating, this is a deliciously satisfying lunch.

SERVES 4

2–3 skinless chicken breasts, about 300g in total
1 tbsp and 1 tsp rapeseed or sunflower oil, plus extra for greasing
1 tsp soy sauce
2 tbsp lime juice (freshly squeezed or bottled)
4 large wholemeal or multi-grain tortilla wraps
100g fresh beansprouts

For the satay sauce:
100g sugar-free crunchy peanut butter
150ml chicken stock
1 tbsp dry sherry
2 tsp soy sauce
2 tbsp lime juice
1cm piece of fresh ginger, peeled and finely grated
2 tsp clear honey
2 spring onions, trimmed and finely chopped
1 tsp chilli sauce
2 tbsp chopped fresh coriander (optional)

1   Trim the chicken breasts if necessary, then place between two sheets of oiled baking paper and gently bash them with a rolling pin to flatten them slightly (this helps them to cook evenly and will tenderise them). Put them in a glass dish.

2   Combine the 1 tbsp of oil with the soy sauce and lime juice. Drizzle over the chicken pieces, turning them to coat evenly. Cover with cling film and leave to marinate in the fridge for 2–4 hours.

3 To make the satay sauce, combine everything except the fresh coriander in a small heavy-based saucepan. Slowly bring to the boil, then half-cover with a pan lid and cook over a very low heat for 10 minutes, stirring regularly until thickened. Remove from the heat and leave until warm (if it thickens too much as it cools, stir in a spoonful or two of boiling water).

4 Meanwhile, pat the chicken breasts dry on kitchen paper. Heat the 1 tsp of oil in a non-stick frying pan and cook the chicken over a high heat for 2 minutes on each side or until lightly browned, then reduce the heat and continue cooking until the chicken is tender and cooked through.

5 Remove the chicken onto a board and cut into thin slices. Warm the tortilla wraps in the microwave for just a few seconds (this will make them more pliable). (Alternatively, wrap them in foil and put them in the oven preheated to 180°C/fan oven 160°C/gas 4 for 10 minutes.) Scatter each tortilla with beansprouts, then top with the chicken slices.

6 Stir the coriander, if using, into the sauce and drizzle over the chicken. Tuck in the two ends of each tortilla, then roll up. Serve straight away.

TIP

You can use smooth peanut butter or almond butter for the sauce, if you prefer. Turkey escalopes make a good alternative to chicken.

Chickpea Scotch Eggs

Instead of traditional sausage meat, these Scotch eggs have a mildly spiced chickpea and olive exterior, so that they can be enjoyed by vegetarians as well as meat eaters. Rather than deep-frying them, they are shallow-fried to minimise the amount of oil you need for cooking.

SERVES 4

7 small or medium eggs, at room temperature
2 × 400g cans chickpeas, drained and rinsed, or 500g cooked chickpeas (page 25)
1 garlic clove, crushed
1 tsp mild chilli powder or a pinch of dried chilli flakes
75g stoned black olives in oil, drained and chopped
3 tbsp chopped fresh coriander
100g fine wholemeal breadcrumbs (see page 24)
oil, for shallow-frying
salt and freshly ground black pepper
some steamed vegetables or salad, to serve

1 Put 6 of the eggs in a saucepan and pour over just enough tepid water to cover. Bring to the boil, then reduce the heat and simmer for 7 minutes. Turn the eggs a few times in the first few minutes of cooking (this will help to make the yolks central when cooked). Remove the eggs from the pan with a slotted spoon and plunge them into a bowl of cold water to cool (this helps to prevent a black ring from forming around the yolk). Peel the eggs when cool enough to handle and pat them dry with kitchen paper.

2 Put the chickpeas in a food processor and blend for about 1 minute or until finely chopped. Add the garlic, chilli, olives, coriander, a little salt (bear in mind that the olives are already salty) and black pepper. Blend again for about 15 seconds, then turn the mixture into a bowl.

3 Lightly beat the remaining egg with a fork and add 1 tbsp to the mixture. Use your hands to mix everything together, then divide into 6 equal portions.

4 Flatten each portion, then wrap around the hard-boiled eggs as evenly as possible. Roll or brush each with the remaining beaten egg, then roll in the breadcrumbs.

5 Heat about 2cm of oil in a heavy frying pan until hot (if you drop in a cube of bread it should begin to sizzle straight away if hot enough), and carefully add the Scotch eggs two at a time. Fry for 4–5 minutes, turning the eggs frequently, until well browned and crisp all over. Remove with a slotted spoon and drain on kitchen paper.

6 Repeat with the remaining eggs, adding a little more oil if needed and keeping the cooked eggs warm in a low oven if you are planning to serve them hot. Cut each egg in half lengthways and serve hot or cold with some steamed vegetables or a salad, allowing 3 halves per person.

TIP

Use parsley instead of coriander, if you prefer, or leave out the herbs and add 3 very finely chopped spring onions instead.

Suitable for vegetarians.

Dips and Dippers

Pulses and vegetables make tasty dips with a great source of fibre, especially when accompanied by more vegetables for dipping or some wholemeal tortilla chips (page 66). This simple, easy-to-prepare snack is surprisingly rich in protein, vitamins and minerals.

SERVES 4

For the lower-fat hummus:
400g can chickpeas, drained and rinsed, or 250g cooked chickpeas (page 25)
3 tbsp tahini
1 garlic clove, crushed
2 tbsp olive oil
juice of 1 lemon
2 tbsp hot water
salt and freshly ground black pepper

For the avocado and watercress dip:
2 ripe avocados
juice of 1 lime
25g watercress, roughly chopped
2 spring onions, sliced
2 sun-dried tomatoes, chopped
100ml natural yogurt

For the vegetable crudités:
2 celery sticks
2 carrots
½ cucumber

1 To make the hummus, put the chickpeas in a food processor and blend for a few seconds until chopped. Add the tahini, garlic, olive oil, lemon juice, hot water and a little salt and pepper. Blend until smooth and creamy, stopping and scraping down the sides of the food processor once or twice. Transfer to a serving bowl, cover with cling film and chill until ready to serve.

2 To make the avocado and watercress dip, halve the avocados and remove the stones, then peel them. Roughly chop the flesh, then put it into a serving bowl and sprinkle with half the lime juice. Mash with a fork until fairly smooth.

3 Put the watercress in a food processor with the remaining lime juice. Add the spring onions and sun-dried tomatoes. Blend until finely chopped, stopping and scraping down the sides of the food processor halfway through.

4 Scrape the watercress mixture into the bowl of mashed avocado, add the yogurt and mix together. Season to taste with salt and pepper. Cover and chill until ready to serve.

5 To make the vegetable crudités, cut the celery, carrots and cucumber into chunky sticks. Arrange on a platter with the bowls of hummus and the avocado and watercress dip, and serve.

TIP

There's no need to wash out the food processor between making the hummus and the avocado and watercress dip; just make sure you scrape it out thoroughly with a spatula.

Suitable for vegetarians. Vegans should use a non-dairy yogurt to make the avocado and watercress dip.

Baked Vegetable Crisps and Tortilla Chips

Oven-baked crisps and tortillas are healthier than ones that are fried and are a delicious high-fibre snack. Use a mandolin, if you have one, to ensure that they are all the same thickness; otherwise you'll need a little time and patience and a large sharp knife to slice the vegetables.

SERVES 6

For the vegetable crisps:
1 large sweet potato, unpeeled, about 250g in total
2 potatoes, unpeeled, about 300g in total
3 beetroot, unpeeled, about 300g in total
3 tbsp rapeseed or sunflower oil
salt

For the tortilla chips:
4 wholemeal or seeded tortillas, about 150g in total

1   Preheat the oven to 200°C/fan oven 180°C/gas 6. Scrub the vegetables and pat dry on kitchen paper. Cut into thin, even slices, about 3mm, using a mandolin, the fine blade on a food processor, or a sharp knife.

2   Put the sweet potato and potatoes in one bowl and the beetroot slices in another (because the red colour of the beetroot will bleed). Drizzle the potato mixture with 2 tbsp of the oil and the beetroot slices with the remaining 1 tbsp oil. Toss the vegetables slices in the oil so that all the pieces are lightly coated.

3 Spread out the vegetable slices on two or three non-stick baking sheets (or baking sheets lined with baking paper). Sprinkle with a little salt, if you like, then bake for 30 minutes, turning frequently and moving the slices around the sheets so that they cook evenly. They should be crisp and the potatoes golden brown. Transfer to a wire rack to cool completely.

4 While the vegetable crisps are cooking, prepare the tortilla chips. Cut each tortilla into triangular wedges using kitchen scissors. Spread out on a large baking sheet.

5 When the vegetable crisps are removed from the oven, lower the temperature to 170°C/fan oven 150°C/gas 3. Bake the tortilla wedges for 12–15 minutes until crisp and lightly browned. Put on a wire rack to cool completely.

TIP

Keep a close watch on the crisps and chips towards the end of cooking as they burn easily. Some will cook quicker than others, so remove any that are ready.

ADD MORE FIBRE

Carrots and other root vegetables can also be made into vegetable crisps. Serve the crisps and chips with high-fibre dips such as hummus (page 64) or tomato salsa (page 74).

Suitable for vegetarians and vegans.

Warm Prawn, Avocado and Wholewheat Couscous Salad

Sometimes adding fibre to your diet is as simple as using a wholegrain or wholemeal version such as bread, pasta or, in this case, wholewheat couscous, which has around double the amount of fibre compared to that of ordinary white couscous.

SERVES 4

200g giant wholewheat couscous
1 litre boiling vegetable stock
2½ tbsp rapeseed or sunflower oil
½ tsp finely grated orange zest
1 tbsp orange juice
1 tbsp walnut oil
1 tsp Dijon mustard
300g cooked peeled prawns
225g red and yellow cherry tomatoes, halved
1 large avocado
50g baby spinach leaves
salt and freshly ground black pepper

1 Rinse the couscous thoroughly in cold water. Pour the stock into a saucepan, add 1 ½ tbsp of the rapeseed oil and bring back to the boil over a medium heat. When it boils rapidly, add the couscous, stir and cover with a lid.

2 Reduce the heat to low and simmer for 6–8 minutes until the couscous has softened but is still slightly firm to the bite. Tip into a sieve and drain off any excess liquid, then put the sieve over the pan and cover with a lid to keep warm.

3 Meanwhile, put the orange zest in a large serving bowl and add the juice, remaining rapeseed oil, walnut oil and mustard, and season with salt and pepper. Whisk together until slightly thickened. Add the prawns and tomatoes. Halve the avocado and remove the stone, then peel and slice. Add the avocado slices to the bowl and gently mix together to coat in the dressing.

4 By now the couscous should be warm but not steaming hot. If necessary, remove the lid from the sieve and let it cool a little more.

5 Add the warm couscous to the bowl and gently mix again, then add the spinach leaves, mix again and serve immediately just as the spinach begins to wilt in the warmth of the couscous.

Variation

For a sharper citrus dressing, use lime zest and juice instead of orange.

ADD MORE FIBRE
Scatter lightly toasted and roughly chopped walnuts over the top of the salad before serving.

Oriental Sprouted Salad

Sprouting your own pulses is surprisingly simple and, as well as adding fibre to the diet, sprouted pulses provide useful amounts of B vitamins and vitamin C. Packets of beansprouts sold in supermarkets are usually mung beans, but most pulses can be sprouted – aduki beans, chickpeas, whole green and brown lentils, and alfalfa seeds are the easiest.

SERVES 4

1 eating apple
50g radishes
1 large carrot
1 celery stick
100g mung beansprouts (see How to Sprout Pulses below)
50g sprouted alfalfa seeds
1 tbsp sesame seeds, preferably toasted

For the dressing:
1 tbsp rapeseed or sunflower oil
1 tsp toasted sesame oil
2 tsp rice wine vinegar or white wine vinegar
2 tsp light soy sauce
2cm piece of root ginger, peeled and grated
freshly ground black pepper

1 To make the dressing, put the oils, vinegar and soy sauce in a bowl. Squeeze out the grated ginger juices into the bowl. Season with a little black pepper and whisk everything together with a fork.

2 Quarter the apple and remove the core. Cut each quarter in half lengthways, then cut each segment crossways into fairly thin slices. Add to the dressing and toss to coat. Top and tail the radishes and slice into rounds. Add them to the dressing and mix to coat (this will stop them from turning brown).

3   Cut the carrot into 5cm lengths. Cut into thin slices, then into fine matchstick strips. Thinly slice the celery.
4   Add the carrot, celery, mung bean and alfalfa sprouts to the bowl and mix everything together to coat evenly. Sprinkle with sesame seeds and serve.

TIP

The salad is a great accompaniment for hot or cold grilled meat or fish or pastries such as quiche. You could turn it into a main meal with the addition of cubes of smoked tofu or pieces of cooked chicken.

HOW TO SPROUT PULSES

- Rinse the pulses in cold water. Put into a large glass jar, fill with water, then cover with a piece of muslin secured with an elastic band. Leave to soak overnight.
- The next day, pour off the water through the muslin. Refill the jar with water through the muslin, shake gently, then drain off the water. Leave the jar on its side with the beans spread out, away from direct sunlight.
- Twice daily, rinse the pulses with water and drain. After a few days, they will begin to sprout.
- When the shoots are at least 1cm long, put the jar in a sunny place (but not too hot). Let them grow for a few more days, rinsing them at least once a day.
- Tip the beansprouts into a sieve and remove any that haven't germinated. They can be used straight away or kept in a plastic bag in the fridge for a day or two.

Suitable for vegetarians and vegans.

Turkey and Cranberry Salad with Barley

Barley is sometimes added to rich meaty casseroles and is also associated with a well-known fruit-squash drink, but it is often overlooked as a grain in its own right. It is a great alternative to rice and contains more protein and fibre weight for weight than brown rice. Pearl barley is polished, which removes the outer bran layer, so pot barley is preferable for this recipe.

SERVES 4

250g pot barley, soaked overnight (see Tip)
50g dried cranberries
250g green beans, trimmed and halved
1 ripe pear
2 tsp lime juice
250g cooked turkey, cut into bite-sized pieces
50g pecan or walnut pieces, lightly toasted (see page 29) and roughly chopped
50g lamb's lettuce or baby salad leaves

For the citrus dressing:
3 tbsp orange juice
1 tsp lime juice
2 tbsp rapeseed or sunflower oil
salt and freshly ground black pepper

1 Drain the soaked barley and tip into a saucepan. Cover with water, bring to the boil, then reduce the heat, half-cover the pan with a lid and simmer for 12–15 minutes until the grains are tender but still firm. Drain well in a colander and leave to cool.

2 While the barley is cooking, put the cranberries in a small bowl and pour over just enough boiling water to cover them. Leave to soak for 15 minutes.

3   Cook the green beans in lightly salted boiling water for 2–3 minutes until just tender. Drain and rinse in cold water to stop them from cooking further and to keep their colour bright.

4   Quarter and core the pear. Cut each quarter in half lengthways, then cut each piece crossways into 1cm thick slices. Toss in the lime juice to prevent the flesh from turning brown.

5   Drain the cranberries, reserving 1 tbsp of the soaking liquid. To make the dressing, whisk together the orange and lime juices, reserved cranberry liquid and the oil. Season with salt and pepper to taste.

6   Put the barley, cranberries, beans, pear, turkey and nuts in a serving bowl and mix together. Drizzle over the dressing and mix again. Add the lettuce leaves and gently mix again. Serve straight away or cover and chill for up to 2 hours.

TIPS

If you can't get hold of pot barley, use pearl barley for this recipe; it doesn't need to be soaked overnight. The salad is best served soon after assembling. If you want to make it several hours in advance, or the night before, leave out the toasted nuts and lettuce leaves and add them just before serving.

Lighter Nachos

Nachos are a popular sharing snack, but bought nacho chips can be high in fat and salt. Making your own with wholemeal tortillas is quick, simple and much better for you.

SERVES 4

1 packet wholemeal tortilla wraps, containing at least 6 individual wraps

1 tbsp rapeseed oil

1 red chilli, halved, seeded and finely chopped

100g mozzarella, grated

2 tbsp crème fraîche

2 tbsp roughly chopped fresh coriander

Avocado and Watercress Dip (page 64), or bought guacamole, to serve

For the tomato salsa:

1 tbsp lime juice

1 tsp rapeseed oil

½ small red onion, finely chopped

4 tomatoes, seeds removed, chopped

salt and freshly ground black pepper

For the beans:

400g can red kidney beans, drained and rinsed, or 250g cooked red kidney beans (page 25)

1 garlic clove, crushed

¼ tsp mild chilli powder

¼ tsp ground cumin

2 tbsp hot water

1   Preheat the oven to 180°C/fan oven 160°C/gas 4. Brush each tortilla with a tiny amount of oil on both sides, then, using kitchen scissors, cut into 12 wedges. Put on baking sheets in a single layer and bake for 8–10 minutes until golden and crisp. Check towards the end of the cooking time and remove any that are cooked to prevent them from over-browning. Put on a wire rack to cool completely.

2   Meanwhile, start to make the salsa. Put the lime juice in a small bowl and add the oil and a little salt and pepper, then whisk together. Add the onion and stir to coat in the dressing. Leave to marinate for a few minutes; this will allow the onion flavour to soften and mellow.

3   Tip the beans into a bowl. Add the garlic, chilli, cumin and hot water. Mash the beans to a thick, roughly textured paste. Season to taste with salt and pepper.

4   Put the tortilla chips in a large ovenproof dish. Spoon the bean mixture in tiny piles over them. Stir the tomatoes into the salsa mixture and spoon this in small piles all over the tortilla chips. Scatter over the chopped chilli and mozzarella cheese. Bake for 5 minutes to heat through.

5   Remove from the oven, drizzle over the crème fraîche and scatter with coriander. Serve straight away with the avocado and watercress dip on the side.

TIP

Use lower-fat versions of crème fraîche and mozzarella cheese if you want to reduce the fat content of this dish.

Suitable for vegetarians. Vegans should use a vegan crème fraîche – Oatly make a good version.

Upside-Down Pizza

We often think of pizzas as unhealthy fast food, but this one has an enriched part-wholemeal base and vegetable topping. A quick-and-easy scone mixture is placed over the vegetables during cooking so that the steam helps it to rise and the top, which will become the base, crisps and browns.

MAKES 4 SMALL OR 2 LARGE SERVINGS

6 baby plum tomatoes, halved lengthways
½ yellow pepper, seeded and sliced
1 small courgette, sliced
5 stoned black olives, halved lengthways
2 tsp olive oil
50g plain wholemeal flour
50g self-raising flour
½ tsp baking powder
15g butter or baking margarine, cut into small cubes
50g mature Cheddar cheese, grated
1 egg
1 tbsp semi-skimmed milk
salt and freshly ground black pepper

1   Preheat the oven to 200°C/fan oven 180°C/gas 6. Line the base of a 20cm round shallow cake tin with baking paper. Put the tomatoes, pepper, courgette and olives in a bowl. Drizzle with the olive oil and season with black pepper. Gently toss the vegetables with your hands to coat in the oil and seasoning. Arrange over the base of the prepared tin, remembering that you will be turning the pizza out upside-down, so whatever is on the bottom of the tin will become the top.

2   Sift the flours, baking powder and a pinch of salt into a mixing bowl, adding the bran left in the sieve. Add the butter and rub in with your fingertips until the mixture resembles fine breadcrumbs. Stir in the grated cheese.

3 Lightly whisk together the egg and milk in a small bowl. Add to the dry ingredients and mix to a soft dough. Roll out on a lightly floured surface to a circle very slightly smaller than the tin. Carefully place on top of the vegetables.

4 Bake for 18–20 minutes until the base is risen and lightly browned. Allow the pizza to stand in the tin for a few minutes before turning out onto a board. Remove the lining paper and cut into wedges to serve.

FOR EXTRA FIBRE

The mixture of wholemeal and white flour gives a light, crisp base. You can use all wholemeal flour if you prefer, in which case add an extra ¼ tsp baking powder and an additional 1 tbsp milk when making the mixture.

Suitable for vegetarians.

Mini Pizza Grills

This pizza-style lunch is quick and easy to make and can be ready to serve in less than 15 minutes. It's worth keeping a packet of wholemeal muffins in the freezer to make these (cut them in half before freezing) – they can then be used straight from frozen.

SERVES 4

4 English wholemeal muffins
25g softened butter or spread
2 tbsp sun-dried tomato paste
½ tsp dried mixed herbs
150g mozzarella cheese, thinly sliced
1 red or yellow pepper, halved, seeded and very thinly sliced
6 cherry tomatoes, halved
6 stoned black or green olives, halved
1 pepperoni salami stick, thinly sliced (optional)

1 Preheat the grill to medium. Cut the muffins in half horizontally using a serrated knife to make 8 halves. Grill the uncut sides for about 1–3 minutes or until browned and crisp, then turn over and grill the cut sides for a little less time, until dry and just starting to brown.

2 Meanwhile, blend the butter with the tomato paste and mixed herbs – don't worry if it doesn't blend completely.

3 Thinly spread the tomato butter over the cut sides of the muffins. Arrange the mozzarella on top, then add the pepper slices, cherry tomatoes and olives (3 halves on each). Top with the pepperoni salami slices if using.

4 Cook under the grill for 4–5 minutes until the cheese is bubbling and the vegetables are tender and lightly browned. Let the pizzas cool for a minute or two before serving.

TIP

You can use ordinary tomato paste if you prefer, but sun-dried tomato paste has a more rounded flavour as it contains rehydrated sun-dried tomatoes, garlic and ground black pepper.

FOR EXTRA FIBRE

Serve the mini pizza grills with a crunchy coleslaw. Put 200g finely shredded white cabbage in a bowl and add 1 large coarsely grated carrot, 1 finely sliced red onion and 2 sliced celery sticks. Add 75g chopped ready-to-eat apricots or raisins, if you like. Mix together, then add 4 tbsp mayonnaise and 3 tbsp natural yogurt, and salt and pepper to taste. Mix well, cover with cling film and chill for several hours if time allows, to let the flavours mingle.

Suitable for vegetarians (leave out the pepperoni or use a vegan version).

Baked Spanish Omelette

Traditionally, Spanish omelette is a simple onion, potato and egg dish cooked on the hob using a large amount of oil, then precariously turned over or finished by browning under the grill. Here, extra vegetables add to the colour, flavour and fibre of the finished dish, which is baked in the oven for easy cooking.

SERVES 4

2 tbsp olive oil
75g frozen peas
1 red onion, sliced
2 potatoes, about 350g, peeled and cut into 1cm dice
1 small red pepper, seeded and cut into 1cm dice
1 garlic clove, crushed
5 medium eggs
100ml semi-skimmed milk
2 tbsp chopped fresh parsley (optional)
salt and freshly ground black pepper

1   Preheat the oven to 180°C/fan oven 160°C/gas 4. Grease the inside of a 20cm round ovenproof dish, preferably non-stick, with 1 tsp of the oil. Spread out the peas on a plate to allow them to start defrosting while you cook the vegetables.

2   Heat the remaining oil in a large non-stick frying pan, add the onion and gently cook over a low heat for 3 minutes, stirring frequently.

3   Turn up the heat a little, add the potatoes and red pepper and cook for a further 3 minutes, then add the garlic and cook for 2–3 minutes, until the potatoes are almost cooked and are beginning to brown. If the vegetables start to stick, sprinkle with a spoonful or two of water and cook until all the liquid has evaporated.

4   Turn off the heat and stir in the peas, then tip the vegetables into the prepared dish and spread them out evenly.

5 Whisk the eggs with the milk and parsley, if using. Season to taste with salt and pepper. Pour over the vegetables. Bake for 25–30 minutes until the top is lightly browned and the omelette softly set. Leave to stand for a minute or two, then loosen the edges and cut into wedges to serve.

TIP

Make use of the oven by baking cookies or a cake at the same time. Peanut Butter Cookies (page 180), Tropical Fruit Malt Teabread (page 172) and Banana and Date Loaf (page 170) are all cooked at the same oven temperature.

FOR EXTRA FIBRE

Slice two tomatoes and arrange on top of the cooked vegetables before pouring over the egg mixture.

Suitable for vegetarians.

Re-Fried Bean Burritos with Fresh Tomato Salsa

Pinto beans, with their pink-and-red speckled skins, have a creamy texture when cooked, which makes them ideal to go with spicy flavours. Although the name of this classic dish suggests otherwise, the beans aren't fried twice; they are gently simmered, then cooked in just a little oil.

SERVES 4

250g dried pinto beans, soaked in cold water for at least 8 hours
2 onions, peeled but left whole
2 garlic cloves, peeled
2 bay leaves
2 tbsp rapeseed or sunflower oil
salt and freshly ground black pepper

For the tomato salsa:
450g firm ripe tomatoes
1 fresh red or green chilli, seeded and finely chopped
finely grated zest and juice of 1 lime
4 tbsp chopped fresh coriander
¼ tsp caster sugar

To serve:
8 large wholemeal or seeded tortillas
50g Monterey Jack or Cheddar cheese, grated
¼ iceburg lettuce, finely shredded
100g Greek-style yogurt

1   Drain the beans and rinse under cold running water. Put them in a large saucepan, cover with plenty of cold water and add one of the onions, cut into quarters, 1 of the garlic cloves and the bay leaves. Bring to the boil and boil rapidly for 10 minutes, then reduce the heat, partly cover the pan with a lid and simmer for 45–50 minutes until the beans are tender.

2   Meanwhile, to make the salsa, chop the tomatoes and put them in a bowl with the chilli, lime zest and juice and the coriander. Sprinkle over the sugar, season with salt and pepper and mix well. Cover and leave at room temperature for the flavours to mingle.

3   When the beans are ready, ladle out and reserve 150ml of the cooking liquid. Drain the beans, discarding the onion quarters, garlic clove and bay leaves.

4   Finely chop the remaining onion and crush the remaining garlic clove. Heat the oil in a large frying pan, add the onion and cook over a medium-low heat for 5 minutes. Add the garlic and cook, stirring frequently for a further 4–5 minutes until soft. Reduce the heat to low. Add a ladleful of the beans and a little of the reserved cooking liquid. Mash with a fork to break up the beans.

5   Continue adding the beans, a ladleful at a time, with some of the cooking liquid, and continue mashing and cooking to make a moist but not wet purée. Season with salt and pepper to taste.

6   Warm the tortillas in the microwave or oven, according to the packet instructions. Spoon the refried beans into the centre of each, sprinkle with a little cheese and top with shredded lettuce and yogurt. Roll up and serve two per person, topped with the tomato salsa. Serve straight away.

FOR EXTRA FIBRE

Serve with some slices or chunks of avocado, tossed in a little lime juice to stop it from browning.

Suitable for vegetarians.

Feta, Black-Eyed Bean and Potato Parcels

These can be served hot or cold, so they are perfect for picnics and packed lunches, or they can be paired with a substantial salad and served as a main meal if you prefer. The sweetness of the dried apricots works well with salty feta cheese, but you could use raisins or sultanas if you prefer.

SERVES 4 (MAKES 8)

200g new potatoes, scrubbed and cut into 1cm dice
4 tbsp olive oil
1 small onion, finely chopped
1 tsp ground cumin
1 tsp ground coriander
50g ready-to-eat dried apricots, chopped
2 × 400g cans black-eyed beans, drained and rinsed, or 500g cooked black-eyed beans (page 25)
50g feta cheese, crumbled
6 stoned green olives in oil, chopped
16 sheets filo pastry about 30 × 18cm each, about 275g in total
2 tsp poppy seeds
salt and freshly ground black pepper

1 Add the potatoes to a pan of lightly salted boiling water. Bring back to the boil, reduce the heat, part-cover the pan with a lid and cook for 5 minutes or until just tender, but still firm. Drain well.

2 Meanwhile, heat 2 tsp of the oil in a non-stick frying pan and gently cook the onion for 6–7 minutes until softened. Stir in the cumin and coriander, cook for a few more seconds, then turn off the heat. Stir in the apricots, black-eyed beans, potatoes, feta and olives, and season with black pepper. Leave to cool.

3 Preheat the oven to 190°C/fan oven 170°C/gas 5. Line a baking sheet with baking paper. Lay a sheet of the pastry on a board or clean work surface and lightly brush with a little of the remaining oil. Top with a second sheet of filo and brush with oil. Spoon one-eighth of the filling on one of the shorter ends, leaving a 3cm gap on each side of the filling from the longer edges.

4 Fold the long sides of the filo pastry (where there is a 3cm gap) over the filling, then roll up to make a parcel. Place seam-side down on the baking sheet. Repeat with remaining pastry sheets, oil and filling mixture to make 8 parcels. Brush the tops with any remaining oil and sprinkle with seeds.

5 Bake for 20–22 minutes until dark golden brown and crisp. Leave to cool on the baking sheet for a few minutes, then carefully remove and serve straight away or put on a wire rack to cool completely.

TIP

Use a good-quality, well-flavoured olive oil for these. If you don't like olive oil, use a slightly nutty flavoured oil such as rapeseed or groundnut, or an almost flavourless oil such as sunflower. You could also use a garlic- or chilli-infused oil.

Suitable for vegetarians.

Classic Kimchi

Along with fibre, fermented foods can help to increase the number of beneficial bacteria in your gut (page 6). Kimchi is an essential part of the Korean diet and provides a combination of salty, sweet, spicy and sour flavours. It's delicious served as an accompaniment to grilled foods, cold meats and cheeses.

MAKES A 1 LITRE JAR

1 small head of Chinese leaves, finely shredded
1 red pepper, quartered, seeded and thinly sliced
1 large carrot, coarsely grated
150g radishes, thinly sliced
2 spring onions, thinly sliced
2.5cm piece of fresh ginger, peeled and grated
15g sea salt flakes
10ml fish sauce
10ml gochugaru (Korean chilli powder, see Tip)
filtered or cooled boiled water, as needed

1 Put all the prepared vegetables in a large clean bowl, add the ginger, then sprinkle over the salt. Gently massage the vegetables with your hands for 5 minutes. The vegetables will feel tough and squeaky at first, but will gradually soften and start to ooze juices. Leave to stand for 5 minutes; the salt will continue to work and extract juices from the vegetables.

2 Sprinkle over the fish sauce and chilli powder, then mix and massage again for 2–3 minutes. You should now have a much-reduced volume of vegetables in their own briny juices.

3 Pack the vegetables and brine into a sterilised, sealable 1 litre glass jar, packing down the vegetables so that they are completely submerged and leaving a 5cm fermenting space at the top of the jar. If there isn't enough liquid, add a little filtered or cooled boiled water to cover.

4   Put on the lid, close firmly, then loosen by a quarter turn. Leave the jar at room temperature out of direct sunlight for seven days. Each day allow any gases to escape by opening the lid, closing it firmly, then loosening it by a quarter turn.
5   Taste after seven days, then every couple of days thereafter, until to your liking; it will get tangier and more fermented with time. Store in the fridge for up to 3 months; the cold will slow down the fermentation to almost nothing, although you should still open the jar now and then to allow the gases to escape.

TIPS

If you can't get gochugaru, use 1 tsp chilli powder (hot or mild, whichever you prefer) and 1 tsp smoked paprika.

When preserving by fermentation, it is essential that everything is clean. Mix the vegetables in a heatproof bowl that has been sterilised (as far as possible) by pouring in boiling water, leaving it for a few minutes, then carefully tipping it away. Chopping boards and other equipment should be very clean (a hot dishwasher is effective) as should be your hands, but don't use anti-bacterial soap or washing-up liquid as these can destroy the beneficial bacteria that you are relying on to start the kimchi fermenting.

Kimchi is fairly salty, but the salt is essential for preventing the growth of harmful bacteria, so don't be tempted to reduce it. You can squeeze out some of the salty brine when serving.

Suitable for vegetarians and vegans, if fish sauce is omitted.

Quinoa Falafels in Wholemeal Pittas

Quinoa has a fantastic nutritional profile when compared to other grains. It contains all nine essential amino acids, making it a good choice for vegans. It is also low in fat and is cholesterol-free. Here, it is combined with chickpeas – also high in protein and fibre – to make tasty little falafels to serve in pittas.

SERVES 4

3 tbsp rapeseed or sunflower oil

1 small onion, finely chopped

1 garlic clove, crushed

65g quinoa

1 tsp ground cumin

1 tsp ground coriander

200ml vegetable stock

400g can chickpeas, drained and rinsed, or 250g cooked chickpeas (page 25)

2 tsp tahini

2 tbsp chopped fresh coriander

quinoa flour, wholemeal flour or plain flour, for dusting

salt and freshly ground black pepper

crunchy coleslaw (see For Extra Fibre on page 79), to serve (if vegan, make with vegan mayonnaise and non-dairy yogurt)

For the wholemeal pittas:

150g wholemeal strong bread flour

100g strong white bread flour, plus extra for dusting

7g sachet easy-blend dried yeast

1 tsp salt

100ml natural yogurt

3 tbsp warm water

1 tbsp olive oil

1   To make the pittas, put the flours in a large bowl, add the yeast and salt, and mix well. Make a hollow in the centre. Put the yogurt in a jug and add the warm water and oil. Stir together, then pour into the hollow. Mix to a soft dough. Knead the dough on a lightly floured surface and knead for 5 minutes, until smooth. Return the dough to the bowl, cover with cling film and leave to rise in a warm place for about 1 hour or until doubled in size.

2   Turn out the dough onto your work surface and knock it back with your knuckles, then divide into 4 pieces. Shape each into a ball, cover with cling film and leave to rest for 10 minutes. Roll out each ball into an oval shape about 18cm long and 5mm thick. Arrange the breads on a greased baking sheet, cover with oiled cling film and leave to rise for 30 minutes.

3   While the pittas are rising, preheat the oven to 230°C/fan oven 210°C/gas 8. Spray or sprinkle the pittas with water (the steam softens them and helps them to rise) and bake for 5 minutes. Transfer to a wire rack and cover with a tea towel to keep them soft.

4   While the pittas are proving and baking, make the falafels. Heat 1 tbsp of the oil in a saucepan and gently cook the onion for 5 minutes or until almost soft. Stir in the garlic, quinoa, cumin and ground coriander, and cook over a low heat for 1 minute. Pour in the vegetable stock, stir, then cover with a lid and cook over a low heat for 20 minutes or until all the stock has been absorbed. Turn off the heat, remove the lid and leave until barely warm.

5   Tip the quinoa mixture into a food processor, add the chickpeas and tahini, and season with salt and pepper. Pulse the food processor until the mixture is blended but not completely smooth. Add the coriander and briefly blend again until mixed.

6 Using your hands, shape the mixture into 16 balls using a little flour, if needed, to stop your hands getting sticky. Heat the remaining 2 tbsp oil in a frying pan and fry the falafels for 5–7 minutes until golden, turning occasionally to ensure even browning (if your frying pan isn't large enough, you might need to do this in two batches). Drain the falafels on kitchen paper. Split open the warm pittas and fill with the falafels and crunchy coleslaw. Serve warm.

Suitable for vegetarians. Vegans should replace the yogurt with a dairy-free yogurt.

Main Meals

If you eat your main meal in the evening, this is a chance to have a large portion of starchy carbohydrates, which can have a calming effect. You should avoid eating too much at your midday meal, however, as they can make you feel a little sluggish. Try to make these wholemeal or wholegrain choices, such as brown rice, wholewheat pasta and couscous, or wholemeal or seeded versions of tortillas, naan bread and pittas. Remember that although meat and fish are great sources of protein and minerals such as iron, they contain no fibre at all, so you need to source this from the ingredients you add to the dish.

Many of the dishes here draw their inspiration from much-loved cuisines from around the world, giving a wide choice of dishes for every occasion. Try Moroccan-Style Chicken and Chickpea Casserole (page 92), Chinese-Spiced Duck with Kumquats (page 102), Beef Jambalaya (page 106) or Mediterranean Lamb and Vegetable Kebabs (page 110).

Vegetarians and vegans have a head start when it comes to fibre intake, as they already value vegetables, pulses, nuts and seeds. Even if you are an avid meat eater, try to make at least one meal a week meat-free.

Moroccan-Style Chicken and Chickpea Casserole

Casseroling is an excellent way to cook inexpensive chicken thighs, as it produces succulent meat and a rich sauce. High-fibre wholewheat couscous is an excellent accompaniment for this simplified, mild version of a classic spicy Moroccan dish.

SERVES 4

6 boneless chicken thighs, skin removed

4 tsp olive oil

2 onions, sliced

2 garlic cloves, crushed

1 tsp chilli powder

1 tsp ground cumin

½ tsp ground cinnamon

400g can chopped tomatoes

300ml vegetable stock

400g can chickpeas, drained and rinsed, or 250g cooked chickpeas (see Tip)

75g soft (no-soak) dried apricots, halved

50g blanched almonds

1 small bunch fresh coriander (about 10g), roughly chopped

a few fresh mint sprigs (about 5g), roughly chopped

salt and freshly ground black pepper

wholewheat couscous with sultanas (optional) and Minted Yogurt (see page 52), to serve

1   Cut the chicken thighs in half and pat them dry with kitchen paper. Heat 2 tsp of the oil in a large non-stick frying pan over a high heat. Add the chicken and cook for about 2 minutes on each side until lightly browned. Remove from the pan and leave to one side.

2 Reduce the heat to low and add the remaining 2 tsp oil. Add the onions and cook for 5 minutes, stirring frequently, then add the garlic and cook for a further 1 minute.

3 Sprinkle over the chilli, cumin and cinnamon. Stir for a few seconds, then add the chopped tomatoes, stock, chickpeas, apricots and almonds. Season with salt and pepper to taste.

4 Bring to the boil, then half-cover the pan with a lid and gently simmer for 25 minutes or until the chicken is tender, stirring occasionally.

5 Stir in the fresh herbs, then turn off the heat and leave to stand for 3 minutes. Serve with wholewheat couscous, tossed with a few sultanas, if you like, and the minted yogurt.

TIP

A 400g can of chickpeas yields about 250g of beans once drained. Dried chickpeas roughly double their weight once cooked, so to get 250g cooked chickpeas you'll need to cook 125g dried chickpeas (see page 25 for the cooking method).

NUTRITIONAL NOTE

Despite its name, the chickpea is not really a pea but a seed. It's a good source of protein for those following a vegetarian diet, and combining chickpeas with dairy foods such as yogurt makes a nutritionally well-balanced dish.

Creamy Chicken, Mushroom and Artichoke Filo Pie

Not all pies are loaded with fat and carbohydrate; they can fit perfectly into a healthy high-fibre diet, too. Deliciously crisp, low-fat filo is scrunched here for an easy pastry topping over a creamy filling of chunks of moist tender chicken and flavourful mushrooms and artichokes.

SERVES 4

2 tsp olive oil, plus extra for brushing
200g baby mushrooms
3 skinless chicken breasts, about 350g, cut into bite-sized chunks
1 bay leaf
150ml dry white wine
200g soft cheese with garlic and herbs
400g can artichoke hearts in water, drained and quartered
4 sheets filo pastry, about 50g
salt and freshly ground black pepper
new potatoes and steamed broccoli or chard to serve

1 Preheat the oven to 200°C/fan oven 180°C/gas 6 and lightly grease a 1.7 litre ovenproof dish. Heat the olive oil in a medium saucepan, preferably non-stick, add the mushrooms and cook for 5 minutes, until lightly browned and tender. Tip the mushrooms and any juices into a bowl and leave to one side.

2 Put the chicken in the saucepan, then add the bay leaf and pour in the wine. Slowly bring to the boil, then reduce the heat and gently simmer, uncovered for 3 minutes (the chicken won't be completely cooked). Lift the chicken out of the pan with a slotted spoon and add to the mushrooms.

3 Bring the wine to a rapid boil and let it bubble for 4–5 minutes so that it reduces slightly. Turn off the heat. Remove the bay leaf and discard. Add the soft cheese to the wine and whisk until blended. Season to taste with salt and pepper. Return the chicken and mushrooms to the pan with the artichokes, and gently mix together. Transfer the mixture to the prepared dish.

4 Lightly brush each sheet of filo pastry, one at a time, with olive oil, then scrunch slightly and put on top of the chicken mixture. Bake on the centre shelf of the oven for 15 minutes, then lower the oven temperature to 180°C/fan oven 160°C/gas 4 and cook for a further 10–15 minutes until the filo is crisp. Serve with new potatoes cooked in their skins and a steamed green vegetable, such as broccoli.

FOR EXTRA FIBRE

Add a handful of frozen peas to the filling (no need to defrost them first), when stirring the chicken and vegetables into the sauce.

One-Pan Roast Chicken with Vegetables

Rather than roasting a whole bird and cooking vegetables separately, here everything is cooked in one pan, which simplifies cooking and saves on washing-up, too! This is a great roast for summer and early autumn when peppers and courgettes are plentiful and inexpensive.

SERVES 4

8 chicken thighs on the bone, skinned
4 tsp olive oil
2 tsp chopped fresh rosemary or thyme
2 red onions, each cut into 8 wedges
2 large sweet potatoes, cut into 3cm chunks
1 red or yellow pepper, seeded and cut into 3cm chunks
2 courgettes, cut into 3cm slices
salt and freshly ground black pepper

1 Preheat the oven to 190°C/fan oven 170°C/gas 5. Remove any excess fat from the chicken and trim if necessary. Arrange in a large roasting tin and brush with 1 tsp of the oil. Sprinkle with the rosemary and season with a little salt and pepper. Cover the tin with foil.

2 Roast the chicken in the oven for 15 minutes. Meanwhile put the onions, sweet potatoes, pepper and courgettes in a large bowl and drizzle over the remaining oil. Mix with your hands so that the vegetables are lightly coated all over with oil.

3   Add the vegetables to the roasting tin, turning them to coat
    in the cooking juices from the chicken. Return the tin to the
    oven (uncovered) and cook for a further 25–30 minutes until
    the chicken is cooked through (pierce the thickest part with
    a skewer – the juices should run clear and not be at all pink),
    and all the vegetables are tender. Turn the vegetables
    halfway through cooking, so that they brown evenly, and if
    they start to colour too much, re-cover the tin with the foil.

4   Let the chicken and vegetables stand for a few minutes to let
    the meat 'rest' (if you like, you can use this time to make a
    quick gravy), then serve on warmed plates, allowing 2
    chicken thighs per person.

TIP

Bake a dessert in the oven at the same time. Oaty Apricot Crumble
(page 138) is cooked at the same temperature.

FOR EXTRA FIBRE

You could also add 2 carrots, cut into 3cm lengths, to the roasted
vegetable mix or serve with an extra green vegetable such as
steamed cabbage.

Cheese-Topped Chicken and Mushroom Enchiladas

Wholewheat tortillas are great for making lunchtime wraps, but they are even better filled with a well-flavoured chicken and vegetable mixture, topped with cheese and baked until golden and crispy. Serve these with a big green salad or coleslaw.

SERVES 4

2 tbsp olive oil
1 tsp lemon juice
3 skinless chicken breasts, cut into strips
1 large onion, finely sliced
1 celery stick, trimmed and thinly sliced
1 garlic clove, crushed
200g brown cap or chestnut mushrooms, chopped
50g sun-dried tomatoes, chopped
50g toasted pine nuts
100g Cheddar cheese, grated
8 wholewheat or seeded flour tortillas
salt and freshly ground black pepper
salad or crunchy coleslaw (see For Extra Fibre on page 99),
   to serve

1 Preheat the oven to 180°C/fan oven 160°C/gas 4. Whisk together 1 tbsp of the oil and the lemon juice in a bowl. Add the chicken strips and toss together to coat. Leave to marinate for a few minutes.

2 Heat the remaining 1 tbsp of oil in a large non-stick frying pan, add the onion and cook for 3 minutes, stirring frequently. Add the celery and garlic, and cook for a further 1 minute, then add the mushrooms and cook for 3 minutes or until the vegetables are almost tender. Stir in the sun-dried tomatoes and pine nuts. Tip the vegetable mixture into a bowl and leave to one side. Wipe the pan clean with kitchen paper.

3 Put the pan over a high heat for a few minutes. Add the chicken and stir-fry for 2–3 minutes until browned and tender. Add to the vegetable mixture and gently mix together, then sprinkle over 50g of the grated cheese, season with a little salt and pepper and mix again.

4 Divide the mixture between the tortillas and roll them up. Put seam-side down (so that they don't unroll) in a large baking dish or roasting tin, then sprinkle with the remaining 50g of cheese.

5 Bake for 20–25 minutes until the tortillas are crisp at the ends and the cheese is golden-brown and bubbling. Divide between four plates, allowing two tortillas per person, and serve straight away with a salad or coleslaw.

FOR EXTRA FIBRE

Serve with a mixed bean salad. Drain and rinse a 400g can mixed beans and mix with 2 finely chopped spring onions and 2 seeded and chopped tomatoes. Whisk 2 tbsp olive oil with 2 tsp white wine vinegar, ½ tsp Dijon mustard, and salt and pepper to taste, and drizzle over the salad. Mix well before serving.

Turkey Meatballs in Tomato Sauce

These tasty turkey meatballs contain grated carrot, which keeps them beautifully moist as they simmer in a rich tomato sauce. Serve them on top of wholewheat spaghetti or pasta shapes for a satisfying meal, or spiralised courgetti if you want a lower-calorie accompaniment.

SERVES 4

1 tbsp olive oil
1 onion, finely chopped
1 garlic clove, crushed
350g minced turkey
25g wholemeal breadcrumbs (page 24)
1 carrot, finely grated
½ tsp dried mixed herbs
1 egg
1 tsp Dijon mustard
salt and freshly ground black pepper

For the tomato sauce:
400g chopped tomatoes
100ml well-flavoured chicken or vegetable stock
2 tsp sun-dried tomato paste
2 tbsp torn or shredded basil leaves or chopped fresh parsley (optional)
300g wholewheat spaghetti
freshly grated Parmesan (optional), to serve

1   Heat the oil in a non-stick frying pan. Add the onion and cook over a low heat for 6–7 minutes, stirring frequently. Add the garlic and cook for a further minute, stirring. Turn off the heat. Spoon a heaped tablespoon of the onion mixture into a bowl. Leave to cool.

2 Add the turkey, breadcrumbs, carrot and dried herbs to the bowl. Whisk the egg with the mustard and add to the bowl. Season with salt and pepper, then mix everything together well with your hands. Roll the mixture into 20 meatballs about the size of a walnut.

3 To make the sauce, put the chopped tomatoes in the frying pan with the onion mixture and add the stock and sun-dried tomato paste, then bring to the boil. Reduce the heat and simmer for 2–3 minutes, stirring occasionally.

4 Add the meatballs to the tomato sauce, cover the pan with a lid and simmer for 10–12 minutes, carefully turning the meatballs over once or twice, so that they cook evenly. Push the meatballs to one side of the pan and stir the basil, if using, into the sauce. Season with salt and pepper.

5 Meanwhile, bring a large pan of boiling, lightly salted water to the boil. Add the spaghetti, half-cover the pan with a lid and simmer for 10–12 minutes until cooked, or according to the pack instructions. Drain thoroughly and divide between four bowls. Top with the meatballs and sauce, and serve with freshly grated Parmesan.

TIP

If you prefer a smooth tomato sauce, purée the chopped tomatoes in a blender before using.

FOR EXTRA FIBRE

Add a celery stick, very finely chopped, to the sauce in step 3.

Chinese-Spiced Duck and Kumquats

Although they look like small oval oranges, the skin of kumquats has a sweet flavour and the whole fruit can be eaten. They complement the richness of the duck in this dish perfectly providing a lovely citrus tang as well as a good amount of fibre.

SERVES 4

2 large boneless duck breasts
1 tsp Chinese five-spice powder
1 tsp ground ginger
2 tbsp rapeseed or sunflower oil
6 shallots, quartered lengthways (see Tip)
4 celery sticks, cut into 2cm slices on the diagonal
12 kumquats, cut into quarters lengthways and pips removed
150g beansprouts
225g can water chestnuts, drained and sliced
200g pak choi, shredded
1 tbsp clear honey
1 tbsp soy sauce
3 tbsp orange juice
3 tbsp well-flavoured vegetable stock
wholewheat noodles or soba noodles, to serve

1   Remove the skin and fat from the duck breasts, then cut across the grain into thin strips. Sprinkle with the five-spice powder and ginger, and toss to coat. Leave to one side while preparing the vegetables.

2   Heat a wok or large non-stick frying pan over a high heat until hot, then add 1 tbsp of the oil and swirl to coat the pan. Add the duck and cook for about 2 minutes, stirring until well-browned (it should still be pink in the centre). Tip out of the pan onto a plate and leave to one side.

3 Add the remaining 1 tbsp oil to the pan and cook the shallots for 2–3 minutes until golden-brown. Reduce the heat to medium-high, add the celery and continue cooking for about 1 minute, then add the kumquats and cook for a further 1 minute.

4 Stir in the beansprouts, water chestnuts and pak choi. Stir-fry for 1 minute until the pak choi is wilted, then reduce the heat to low. Put the honey in a small bowl and add the soy sauce, orange juice and stock, then mix together. Add to the pan, then stir in the duck and let the mixture bubble for 1–2 minutes until the sauce has thickened. Serve straight away in warmed bowls on a bed of wholewheat or soba noodles.

TIP

To peel the shallots, put them in a heatproof bowl and pour over enough boiling water to cover. Leave for 3 minutes, then drain. When cool enough to handle, the skins should be easy to remove and the shallots slightly softened.

FOR EXTRA FIBRE

Add some chopped toasted cashew nuts or sesame seeds at the end of cooking. Don't discard the leaves from the celery. Tear these into smaller pieces and scatter them over the top of the dish as a garnish.

Duck and Mixed Mushroom Risotto

Although white rice itself has little fibre, you can still enjoy creamy and rich risottos. The fibre source in this dish comes from the generous amount of mushrooms and beans it contains. Risottos do take up quite a lot of time simply stirring, but they are very easy to make. Keep the stock simmering in a small saucepan while you make the risotto so that you're not adding cool stock to the rice, which would slow down the cooking.

SERVES 4

10g dried porcini mushrooms
1 bay leaf
250ml boiling water
2 tbsp sunflower oil
2 duck breasts, skinned
25g unsalted butter
1 onion, finely chopped
1 garlic clove, crushed
350g risotto rice
150ml dry white wine
finely grated zest of 1 lemon
750ml simmering vegetable or chicken stock
400g can borlotti beans, drained and rinsed, or 250g cooked borlotti beans (page 25)
400g mixed fresh mushrooms, such as chestnut, shiitake and oyster, sliced
3 tbsp chopped fresh parsley
salt and freshly ground black pepper

1 Put the porcini mushrooms in a heatproof bowl with the bay leaf and pour over the boiling water. Leave to soak for 15–20 minutes, then drain, reserving the soaking liquid (tip away the last little bit if there is any grit in it). Finely chop the mushrooms and leave to one side.

2   Meanwhile, heat a heavy frying pan over a high heat until
    hot. Add 1 tbsp of the oil and swirl around the base of the
    pan. Add the duck breasts and reduce the heat to medium.
    Cook for 10 minutes (a little less if you like your duck rare,
    and a little more if you prefer it well done), turning over
    halfway through the cooking time. Remove the duck and
    leave to rest in a warm place.
3   Meanwhile, heat 1 tsp of the remaining oil and 15g of the
    butter in a large saucepan. Add the onion and cook for 5
    minutes over a low heat until softening. Add the garlic and
    cook for a further 1 minute, stirring constantly. Add the rice
    and stir to coat in the butter and oil.
4   Pour in the wine and let it bubble, stirring until it has almost
    evaporated. Stir in the lemon zest and porcini mushrooms and
    liquid. Let it cook, stirring frequently with a wooden spoon
    until the liquid has been absorbed by the rice. Add the stock a
    ladleful at a time, stirring until it has all been absorbed.
    Continue using up the stock in this way, adding the beans with
    the last ladle of stock. Cooking will take 15–20 minutes; the
    risotto is cooked when the rice is still firm but completely
    tender and the texture creamy. When it is ready, take it off the
    heat, cover the pan with a lid and leave to stand for 5 minutes.
5   Meanwhile, heat the remaining 10g butter and 2 tsp oil in the
    frying pan and cook the fresh mushrooms over a high heat
    for 4–5 minutes until tender. Cut the duck into thin slices
    and stir into the risotto with the mushrooms and any juices
    and the parsley. Season to taste with salt and pepper and
    serve in warmed bowls.

FOR EXTRA FIBRE

Add 100g frozen peas, preferably defrosted, with the last ladleful of
stock.

Beef Jambalaya

In this Cajun classic, tender beef and spicy chorizo sausage are cooked in a peppery tomato sauce with vegetables and rice. Although usually made with white rice, the jambalaya works well here using brown basmati rice, which gives the dish a lovely nutty flavour.

SERVES 4

300g rump or sirloin steak

2 tsp mild chilli powder

1 tbsp rapeseed or sunflower oil

150g chorizo sausages, cut into 1cm dice

1 onion, chopped

2 celery sticks, chopped

2 red peppers, seeded and cut into strips

300g brown basmati rice, rinsed

200g can red kidney beans, drained and rinsed, or 125g
   cooked red kidney beans (page 25)

1 tsp ground ginger

2 tsp Cajun seasoning

1 tbsp sun-dried tomato paste

900ml beef or vegetable stock

salt and freshly ground black pepper

1   Trim any fat from the steak, then cut the meat across the grain into thin strips. Sprinkle over the chilli powder on both sides as evenly as possible.

2   Heat the oil in a large non-stick frying pan or wok, add the steak and cook over a high heat for 2–3 minutes until browned but still slightly pink in the centre. Remove from the pan and leave to one side. Add the chorizo and cook for 2–3 minutes until lightly browned. Remove from the pan with a slotted spoon, leaving the oil behind (some will have come out of the chorizo).

3   Reduce the heat to low. Add the onion to the pan and cook for 5 minutes, stirring frequently until golden. Add the celery and peppers and continue cooking for a further 2 minutes. Stir in the rice, beans, ginger, Cajun seasoning and tomato paste. Cook for a further 1 minute, stirring.

4   Pour in the stock and season with salt and pepper. Bring to the boil, reduce the heat, then cover and simmer for about 20 minutes, stirring occasionally, until the rice is tender and most of the liquid absorbed.

5   Return the beef and chorizo to the pan and gently stir over a low heat for 1 minute. Re-cover the pan, turn off the heat and leave to stand for a few minutes. Spoon into warmed bowls and serve straight away.

Variation

Jambalaya is often made with chicken and seafood. Instead of steak, cook 2 large diced skinless chicken breasts, cut into 2cm chunks in step 2, frying them for 4–5 minutes until lightly browned and cooked through. Add 150g large cooked and peeled prawns at step 5.

Updated Cottage Pie

This traditional family favourite is given a healthy update with the addition of lots of vegetables and red lentils. The latter cook down to make a delicious rich and thick sauce. It's then topped with a generous layer of mashed potatoes and swede. Serve with baked beans or peas to add extra fibre.

SERVES 4

3 tsp rapeseed or sunflower oil
450g lean minced beef
1 large onion, finely chopped
2 leeks, finely chopped
2 carrots, finely chopped
2 celery sticks, finely chopped
100g red lentils
3 tbsp tomato purée
1 tbsp Worcestershire sauce
350ml hot beef stock
salt and freshly ground black pepper
baked beans or peas to serve

For the topping:
450g floury potatoes, peeled and cut into chunks
350g swede, peeled and cut into chunks
4 tbsp semi-skimmed milk
15g butter

1   Heat 1 tsp of the oil in a large heavy-based saucepan. Add the beef and cook over a high heat, stirring with a wooden spoon to break up the meat into small pieces, for 4–5 minutes until well browned. Reduce the heat to medium and transfer the meat to a bowl using a slotted spoon.

2   Add the remaining 2 tsp oil to the pan. Add the onion and leeks to the pan and cook for 3–4 minutes until beginning to soften. Add the carrots and celery, and cook for a further 3 minutes, stirring frequently. Return the minced beef to the pan. Stir in the lentils, tomato purée, Worcestershire sauce and stock. Season with salt and pepper, bring to the boil, then reduce the heat, half-cover the pan with a lid and gently simmer for 20 minutes.

3   Meanwhile, to make the topping, put the potatoes and swede in a saucepan and pour over just enough boiling water to cover them. Bring back to the boil, then reduce the heat, cover the pan and simmer for 15–20 minutes until the vegetables are just tender.

4   Preheat the oven to 200°C/fan oven 180°C/gas 6. Drain the potatoes and swede well, then return them to the pan. Mash with the milk until smooth, then add the butter, season with salt and pepper and beat with a wooden spoon until fluffy.

5   Spoon the meat mixture into a large ovenproof dish, about 2.5 litres capacity. Top with the mashed potato and swede mixture, spreading it out evenly. Bake for 20 minutes, until the top is golden brown and the meat sauce is bubbling. Serve with baked beans or peas.

Variation

For a shepherd's pie use 450g lean minced lamb instead of the beef and use parsnips instead of swede in the topping.

Mediterranean Lamb and Vegetable Kebabs

Marinating not only flavours the meat but it also helps to tenderise it, so you need to plan ahead with this recipe and start preparation at least 4 hours before cooking and preferably even longer. You can use bottled lemon juice here, but fresh will taste much better.

SERVES 4

1 tbsp olive oil, plus extra for greasing
juice of 1 large lemon (about 3 tbsp)
1 tbsp chopped fresh mint
½ tsp ground cumin
400g boneless lamb leg or fillet, trimmed and cut into 2.5cm chunks
2 red or yellow peppers, seeded and cut into 4cm chunks
2 medium courgettes, cut into 2cm slices
salt and freshly ground black pepper

For the tzatziki:
½ cucumber
a large pinch of salt
6 tbsp Greek-style yogurt
2 tbsp chopped fresh mint

For the couscous:
200g wholewheat couscous
250ml boiling vegetable stock
2 tbsp pesto

1   Put the oil in a shallow bowl and add the lemon juice, mint, cumin and a little black pepper. Whisk together. Take out 1 tbsp of this marinade and put it into a small bowl. Add the lamb pieces to the shallow bowl and stir to coat in the marinade. Cover with cling film and leave in the fridge for at least 4 hours and up to 24 hours.

2   For the tzatziki, coarsely grate the cucumber and put it in a plastic or stainless steel sieve over a bowl to catch the drips. Sprinkle with the salt. Leave for 15 minutes, then squeeze out the briny juices and discard. Put the cucumber in a bowl, add the yogurt and the mint, and mix well. Chill in the fridge until needed.

3   Bring a pan of lightly salted water to the boil. Add the pepper chunks and cook for 30 seconds, then add the courgettes. Bring back to the boil and simmer for 30 seconds. Drain well. Tip into a bowl, then drizzle over the reserved marinade and toss together to lightly coat.

4   When ready to cook, preheat the grill to high and line the grill pan with foil. Thread the lamb and vegetables on to eight metal kebab skewers; don't pack them too tightly or they won't cook properly.

5   Grill the kebabs for 1 minute on each side, then reduce the heat to medium and cook for a further 5 minutes on each side or until well-browned and tender.

6   Meanwhile, put the couscous in a heatproof bowl and pour over the vegetable stock. Cover the bowl with a pan lid and leave for 10 minutes or until all the stock has been absorbed. Stir in the pesto and fluff up the couscous with a fork. Pile the couscous onto warmed plates, top each with 2 kebabs and serve with a large spoonful of tzatziki.

FOR EXTRA FIBRE

Add 4 chopped sun-dried tomatoes when soaking the couscous and stir in 2 tbsp toasted pine nuts just before serving.

Lamb Tagine

Morocco's hearty tagines are renowned for their succulent meat cooked with tender dried fruit, honey and fragrant spices. They are often served with fresh, crunchy salads, as suggested here, and flatbread, or you could serve with wholegrain couscous (page 110) if you prefer.

SERVES 4

350g stoned dried prunes or a mixture of prunes and ready-to-eat apricots
2 tbsp rapeseed or sunflower oil
400g boned lean lamb, trimmed and cut into 2cm cubes
1 large onion, thinly sliced
1 garlic clove, crushed
1 tbsp ras-el-hanout (see Tip)
400ml lamb or mild beef stock
200g butternut squash, cut into 2cm cubes
400g can chopped tomatoes
finely grated zest of 1 lemon and juice of ½ lemon
1 tbsp clear honey
50g blanched almonds
3 tbsp chopped fresh coriander
salt and freshly ground black pepper
wholemeal flatbreads, to serve (optional)

For the salad:
juice of ½ lemon
2 tbsp olive oil
1 red onion, chopped
1 green pepper, seeded and chopped
2 celery sticks, chopped
3 tbsp chopped fresh mint

1 Preheat the oven to 170°C/fan oven 150°C/gas 3. Put the dried fruit in a heatproof bowl and pour over enough cold water to cover. Leave to soak for a few minutes.

2   Heat 1 tbsp of the oil in a large non-stick frying pan and cook
    the lamb over a high heat for 2–3 minutes, stirring
    frequently, until well browned. Remove from the pan and
    leave to one side.

3   Heat the remaining 1 tbsp oil in the pan, add the onion and
    cook over a medium heat for 5–6 minutes until beginning to
    brown. Add the garlic and cook for 30 seconds, stirring. Add
    the ras-el-hanout and cook for a further 30 seconds.

4   Pour in the stock, then turn off the heat. Stir well, then tip
    the mixture into an ovenproof dish. Add the lamb and any
    juices, the butternut squash, tomatoes, lemon zest and juice,
    honey and almonds.

5   Drain the dried fruit and add to the dish. Stir again. Cover
    with a lid and cook in the oven for 1½–2 hours until the
    lamb is very tender.

6   Meanwhile, to make the salad, whisk the lemon juice and oil
    together in a serving bowl. Add the onion and stir to coat.
    Cover and leave for 1 hour to marinate (this mellows the
    flavour of the onion). Add the remaining salad ingredients and
    season with a little salt and pepper to taste. Stir the chopped
    coriander into the lamb tagine and season to taste with salt.
    Serve with the salad and wholemeal flatbreads, if you like.

TIP

Ras-el-hanout is available in most supermarkets. If you can't find it
or you prefer to make your own, here's how. Put 2 tbsp cumin seed,
2 tbsp coriander seed and the seeds from 10 cardamom pods in a
small non-stick frying pan and toast over a low heat for 3 minutes,
shaking the pan frequently. Add 2 tsp black peppercorns and continue
to toast until aromatic and a slightly darker colour. Leave to cool,
then grind in a spice grinder or using a pestle and mortar, adding a
pinch of saffron strands if you like. Mix with 1 tbsp ground cinnamon,
2 tsp ground ginger and 1 tsp ground turmeric. Store in a small jar.

Sweet and Spicy Stir-Fried Pork

Delicious and healthy, stir-fries are a great way to combine a relatively small amount of meat with lots of high-fibre vegetables. Quick cooking retains most of the nutritional benefits of the ingredients, especially the vitamins, and only a minimal amount of oil is needed.

SERVES 4

300g piece pork fillet
2 tsp toasted sesame oil
1 tbsp lime juice (or 2 tsp lemon juice and 1 tsp water)
2 tbsp soy sauce
1 tbsp groundnut or rapeseed oil
6 spring onions, trimmed and cut into 3cm lengths
1 red pepper, seeded and cut into thick matchsticks
100g broccoli, cut into small florets
100g mangetouts or sugar snap peas, trimmed
300g beansprouts (see page 71)
1 tbsp honey
2 tbsp rice wine or dry sherry or extra vegetable stock
2 tbsp hoisin sauce
1 small mild red chilli, halved, seeded and very finely chopped
3cm piece fresh ginger, peeled and grated
100ml vegetable stock
wholegrain rice or wholewheat egg noodles, to serve

1   Trim any visible fat from the pork. Cut into thick slices, then cut each slice into thick matchstick strips. Put the toasted sesame oil in a bowl and add the lime juice and 1 tbsp of the soy sauce, then whisk together. Add the pork and mix well. Leave to marinate for a few minutes while preparing the vegetables.

2   Heat 1 tsp of the groundnut oil in a large non-stick frying pan or wok. Add the pork strips and stir-fry over a high heat for about 3 minutes; the pork should be well browned and almost cooked through. Remove and leave to one side.

3   Heat the remaining 2 tsp of oil in the pan. Add the spring onions, red pepper and broccoli, and cook for 2 minutes over a high heat, stirring frequently.

4   Reduce the heat a little to medium high, add the mangetouts and cook for 1 minute, stirring, then add the beansprouts and cook for a further 2 minutes. Return the pork and any juices to the pan.

5   Sir the remaining 1 tbsp soy sauce, the honey, rice wine, hoisin sauce, chilli and ginger into the stock. Pour into the pan and cook for 2–3 minutes, stirring continuously, until the pork and all vegetables are cooked. Spoon onto warmed plates or bowls on a bed of rice or noodles and serve.

Variations

- Use whatever vegetables are in your fridge or are seasonal. Courgettes, carrots, baby sweetcorn and mushrooms are just a few of the vegetables that could be added or substituted in this recipe.

- You could also use tender beef steak, such as rump or sirloin, or a couple of chicken breasts instead of the pork.

Smoked Salmon and Asparagus Quiche with a Spelt and Sesame Crust

Instead of traditional shortcrust pastry, the crust for this quiche is made with toasted sesame seeds and wholemeal spelt flour, which gives it a lovely nutty flavour. High-fibre asparagus and salmon are a classic combination and here they are baked in a creamy savoury egg custard.

SERVES 4

150g slender asparagus spears, cut in half

3 eggs

150ml crème fraîche

100ml milk

2 tbsp Pecorino cheese (see Tip) or mature Cheddar, finely grated

50g frozen peas, defrosted

100g smoked salmon trimmings or slices torn into small pieces

freshly ground black pepper

For the spelt and sesame crust:

3 tbsp sesame seeds

175g wholemeal spelt flour

75g butter, cut into small cubes

1 egg, lightly beaten

1   To make the crust, toast the sesame seeds in a dry frying pan over a medium heat until they smell nutty and are just beginning to turn golden. Tip them onto a plate, leave to cool for a few minutes, then transfer them to a large bowl.

2   Add the flour, then rub in the butter using your fingertips until the mixture resembles fine breadcrumbs. Add the egg and stir together to make a firm dough. Roll out the pastry and use to line a 23cm fluted flan tin, trimming off any excess with a sharp knife. Chill in the fridge for 10 minutes.

3   Put a baking sheet in the oven and preheat to 200°C/fan oven 180°C/gas 6. Put the stalk halves of the asparagus in a steamer above a pan of boiling water and steam for 1 ½ minutes. Add the asparagus tips and steam for a further 1 ½ minutes or until they are just beginning to soften. Remove and leave to one side.

4   Prick the quiche case all over with a fork. Line the base and sides with a sheet of baking paper or foil, then weight down with dried beans or ceramic baking beans. Bake on the hot baking sheet for 15 minutes, remove the paper or foil and beans and return to the oven for a further 5 minutes.

5   Put the eggs in a small bowl and beat them lightly using a fork. Season with black pepper. Pour the crème fraîche and milk into a jug and heat in the microwave for 1 minute until warm, but not boiling. (Alternatively, pour into a saucepan and heat gently.) Pour over the eggs, whisking well.

7   Working quickly, scatter the cheese over the base of the quiche case, followed by the peas. Arrange the asparagus and salmon slices on top. Pour over the egg mixture and bake for 5 minutes, then reduce the oven temperature to 180°C/fan oven 160°C/gas 4 and bake for a further 20 minutes or until the filling is lightly set. Leave to cool for 5 minutes, then remove from the tin and serve.

TIP

Pecorino cheese is extremely salty, so don't be tempted to use more than 2 tbsp.

Glazed Cod with Fresh Tomato Dressing

An easy way to add fibre to any dish is to serve it with a fresh vegetable sauce or dressing and, when in season and plentiful, tomatoes are an excellent choice. This dressing also works well with other grilled or barbecued fish and meats such as chicken.

SERVES 4
2 tsp soy sauce
¼ tsp ground ginger
1 tbsp light muscovado sugar
finely grated zest and juice of 1 lime
4 thick cod steaks, with skin, each about 175g
salt and freshly ground black pepper
steamed vegetables, to serve

For the fresh tomato dressing:
450g tomatoes, seeded and chopped (see Tip)
1 tbsp balsamic vinegar
1 tsp light muscovado sugar
4 tbsp olive oil
1 green or red chilli, seeded and finely chopped

1 To make the dressing, put the tomatoes in a blender or food processor with the balsamic vinegar and sugar. Pulse for about 30 seconds until finely chopped.
2 With the motor running, gradually add the olive oil in a slow drizzle. Add the chilli, and season with salt and pepper, then blend for a few more seconds.
3 Put the soy sauce in a bowl and add the ginger, sugar, lime zest and juice, then mix together. Preheat the grill to high, line the grill pan with foil and arrange the fish on it skin-side up. Grill for 2 minutes, then turn the fish over and grill the top for 2 minutes.

4 Brush the glaze over the top and sides of the cod steaks, then grill for a further 2–3 minutes until the glaze is bubbling and the fish is cooked through (the time will depend on the thickness of the fish).

5 Transfer the fish to warmed plates and spoon over the tomato dressing. Serve with steamed fresh vegetables.

TIP

It's better to leave the skins on the tomatoes because they contain a good amount of fibre. You can remove them if you prefer, however: just put them in a heatproof bowl and pour over boiling water to cover. Leave for 1–2 minutes, then drain and rinse under cold water; the skins should slide off easily.

Melting-Middle Fishcakes

These oven-baked fishcakes include tinned tuna and sweetcorn, both useful ingredients to keep in your food cupboard. They have a crisp wholemeal breadcrumb and sesame seed coating and a creamy melting centre flavoured with fresh lemon zest and herbs.

SERVES 4

2 tbsp cream cheese
1 tbsp mayonnaise
2 tsp chopped fresh herbs, such as chives or parsley
finely grated zest of 1 lemon
400g potatoes, cut into large chunks (see Tip)
145g can tuna in oil, drained
200g can sweetcorn, drained
40g fresh wholemeal breadcrumbs
1 tsp rapeseed or sunflower oil
1 tbsp sesame seeds
1 small or medium egg, lightly beaten
salt and freshly ground black pepper
steamed fresh vegetables or salad, to serve

1   Put the cream cheese in a small bowl and add the mayonnaise, herbs and lemon zest, then mix together. Spoon into four ice-cube tray sections and freeze for at least 4 hours or until solid.

2   Cook the potatoes in lightly salted boiling water for 15 minutes or until tender. Drain well and mash until smooth. Season with pepper to taste. Break up the tuna into small chunks and flakes, then stir into the potatoes with the sweetcorn. Leave the mixture until cool.

3 Preheat the oven to 200°C/fan oven 180°C/gas 6. Line a baking tray with baking paper. Turn out the frozen cream cheese mixture from the ice-cube tray, but keep the cubes in the freezer until ready to use.

4 Mix the breadcrumbs with the oil, then mix in the sesame seeds. Divide the potato mixture into four equal portions and, with lightly floured hands, pat out each to a round roughly 12cm in diameter. Put a frozen cream-cheese cube in the centre of each and fold over the edges of the potato to enclose it, shaping it into a fishcake about 9cm across.

5 Dip the fishcakes, one at a time into the beaten egg, then into the breadcrumb mixture to coat them. Place on the baking sheet and cook for 15 minutes or until the outside is crisp and lightly browned. Check that they are cooked through by inserting a skewer into the centre; it should be fairly hot when removed. Serve the fishcakes with steamed fresh vegetables or a salad.

TIP

You can used leftover mashed potato to make these, providing it doesn't contain too much milk and butter, which might make the mixture too soft to handle. You will need 350g.

Fresh Tuna Niçoise

In this French-style salad, fresh tuna steaks are quickly grilled and sliced to serve on top of a colourful mixture of warm and cold vegetables in a herby Dijon mustard dressing. Serve with slices of warm, crusty wholemeal baguette.

SERVES 4

400g small new potatoes, scrubbed
200g French beans, trimmed and halved
150g shelled broad beans, fresh or frozen
2 tuna steaks, each about 200g
olive oil, for brushing
3 Little Gem lettuces, separated into leaves and torn into
   smaller pieces
150g baby plum tomatoes, halved
¼ cucumber, cut into 1cm chunks
75g black olives, stoned
salt and freshly ground black pepper
slices of warm, crusty wholemeal baguette, to serve
   (optional)

For the dressing:
2 tbsp olive oil
1 tbsp red wine vinegar
1 tsp Dijon mustard
2 tbsp roughly torn flat-leaf parsley

1 Put the potatoes in a pan of boiling lightly salted water, bring back to the boil, cover the pan with a lid and cook for 10 minutes. Add the French and broad beans and cook for a further 5 minutes or until all the vegetables are just tender. Drain in a colander and rinse with cold water for just a few seconds to cool slightly and stop them cooking further.

2   Pat the tuna steaks dry with kitchen paper. Lightly brush both sides with oil and sprinkle with salt and pepper. Heat a ridged griddle or non-stick frying pan until hot. Cook the tuna steaks for 2 minutes on each side; the tuna will still be pink in the centre, so cook it for a little longer if you prefer it slightly more done, but take care not to over-cook it or it will be tough and dry. Remove from the pan and put on a plate. Leave to rest for a few minutes.

3   Meanwhile, to make the dressing, put the oil in a screw-top jar and add the vinegar, mustard and 2 tbsp water, then shake together until blended. Add the parsley and briefly shake again.

4   Arrange the lettuce leaves on a platter or individual plates. Tip the potatoes and beans into a bowl and add the tomatoes, cucumber and olives. Drizzle over the dressing, then gently mix together. Put on top of the lettuce leaves.

5   Cut the tuna into slices about 5cm thick. Arrange on top of the potato mixture and serve straight away with slices of wholemeal baguette, if you like.

FOR EXTRA FIBRE

Add a small, ripe avocado, halved, stone removed, peeled and cut into 2cm chunks.

Cauliflower and Chickpea Burgers

When you roast cauliflower it gives it a wonderful nutty flavour, completely different from when it is boiled. Here it is combined with caramelised roasted onions, chickpeas and wholemeal breadcrumbs to make tasty vegetarian burgers. Serve these in wholemeal buns with plenty of salad for a high-fibre meal. Sweet potato chips make a great accompaniment.

SERVES 4

1 small cauliflower, cut into florets
1 onion, sliced
2 tbsp rapeseed or sunflower oil
1 garlic clove, unpeeled and left whole
400g tin chickpeas, drained and rinsed, or 250g cooked
   chickpeas (see page 25)
1½ tsp smoked paprika
½ tsp dried mixed herbs
2 eggs, lightly beaten
50g wholemeal breadcrumbs
flour, for dusting
salt and freshly ground black pepper
4 wholemeal or brown burger buns
lettuce, cucumber, sliced tomatoes and relish or Tzatziki
   (page 110) (optional), to serve

1 Put a non-stick baking tray in the oven and preheat to 200°C/fan oven 180°C/gas 6. Put the cauliflower in a bowl with the sliced onion. Drizzle over 1 tbsp of the oil and toss the vegetables together to coat.

2 Tip the vegetables onto the hot baking tray. Add the whole garlic clove and roast for 15–20 minutes until the vegetables are tender and lightly browned. Turn once or twice during cooking so that they brown evenly. Remove from the oven and leave on the tray to cool for about 10 minutes.

3 Transfer the vegetables to a food processor, squeeze out the roasted garlic from its papery skin, add the chickpeas and process for a minute until chopped. Scrape down the sides, add the paprika and herbs, and season with salt and pepper. Add the eggs and process for a further minute until the chickpea mixture is finely chopped. Scrape down the sides again, add the breadcrumbs and process until combined. The mixture should still have texture with visible pieces of cauliflower and not be a purée.

4 With lightly floured hands, shape the mixture into four burgers. Put on a plate lined with baking paper, cover with cling film and chill until ready to cook.

5 Heat the remaining 1 tbsp oil in a non-stick frying pan over a medium heat. Add the burgers, reduce the heat a little and cook for 5 minutes on each side until browned.

6 Meanwhile, split the burger buns in half and fill with lettuce, cucumber and tomato slices. Add the cooked burgers and top each with the bun lid. Serve straight away with relish, if you like, such as a high-fibre sweetcorn relish or a spoonful or two of tzatziki.

Variation

Fresh herbs are also good in these instead of dried. Try adding 2 tbsp chopped fresh parsley or, for a different flavour, add 1 tsp ground cumin and ½ tsp ground coriander to the mixture instead of paprika and 2 tbsp chopped fresh coriander.

TIP

The burgers can be frozen after cooking. Fry for just 3 minutes on each side until lightly browned, then allow to cool. Wrap individually and freeze for up to 3 months. Defrost in the fridge overnight and re-heat over a low heat in a non-stick frying pan.

Suitable for vegetarians. Vegans should use an egg substitute.

Goat's Cheese and Lentil Nut Loaf

Tangy goat's cheese adds a distinctive flavour to this protein-packed vegetarian loaf. It can be served hot or cold with steamed fresh vegetables or for a lighter meal with a simple salad.

SERVES 4

1 tbsp rapeseed or olive oil, plus extra for greasing
2 leeks, very finely sliced
1 garlic clove, crushed
1 large carrot, coarsely grated
175g red lentils
400ml boiling vegetable stock
1 bay leaf
50g shelled Brazil nuts, coarsely chopped
100g unsalted peanuts or blanched almonds, coarsely
    chopped
40g fresh wholemeal breadcrumbs
3 tbsp chopped fresh parsley
1 egg, lightly beaten
100g firm, crumbly goat's cheese (see Tip)
salt and freshly ground black pepper
steamed vegetables or a salad, to serve

1   Heat the oil in a large non-stick saucepan and gently cook
    the leeks for 5–6 minutes until soft, stirring frequently. Add
    the garlic and cook for a further 1 minute, stirring, then add
    the carrot.
2   Rinse the lentils in a sieve under cold running water. Add to
    the pan with the stock and bay leaf. Slowly bring to the boil,
    then cover with a lid and simmer very gently for 20 minutes
    or until all the stock has been absorbed. Stir frequently
    towards the end of the cooking time, to prevent sticking.
    Remove the lid and allow to cool for 10 minutes, stirring
    occasionally.

3   Meanwhile, toast the Brazil nuts and peanuts in a non-stick frying pan over a low heat until they are just beginning to turn golden and smell nutty. Tip them onto a small plate to stop them cooking further (they burn very easily). Leave to cool. Meanwhile, preheat the oven to 190°C/fan oven 170°C/gas 5. Lightly grease and line a 900g loaf tin with baking paper.

4   Stir the nuts, breadcrumbs and parsley into the lentil mixture and season to taste with salt and pepper, then stir in the beaten egg. Crumble the cheese into small pieces and gently stir into the mixture. Spoon the mixture into the prepared tin and cover loosely with foil.

5   Bake for 45 minutes or until the loaf is firm, removing the foil 20 minutes before the end of cooking time to allow the top to brown. Leave in the tin for 10 minutes, then turn the loaf out onto a board. Serve hot or cold in slices with steamed vegetables.

TIP

Choose a crumbly, rather than spreadable, goat's cheese. Feta cheese makes a good alternative if you want a less distinctively flavoured cheese. Taste the cheese before seasoning the loaf, as some have a high salt content, so you might need to reduce the amount of salt when seasoning the mixture.

Suitable for vegetarians.

Cheese and Potato Slice

This inexpensive dish is cooked in a round tin and cut into wedges to serve. It makes a good midweek meal served with coleslaw and grilled or fried mushrooms and tomatoes. Use a mature Cheddar for the best flavour.

SERVES 4

1 tbsp rapeseed or sunflower oil
2 onions, very thinly sliced
1 garlic clove, crushed
1 tsp vegetable extract
250g porridge (rolled) oats
1 potato, about 175g, thinly sliced
100g mature Cheddar cheese, grated
2 tbsp chopped fresh parsley
2 eggs, lightly beaten
salt and freshly ground black pepper
apple and fennel salad (see For Extra Fibre) and grilled or
    fried mushrooms and tomatoes, to serve

1   Preheat the oven to 180°C/fan oven 160°C/gas 4. Lightly grease and line the base of a 20cm round shallow tin with baking paper. Heat the oil in a large non-stick pan, add the onions and gently fry for 6–7 minutes until tender, stirring occasionally.
2   Add the garlic and cook for a further minute, then add the vegetable extract and 1 tbsp water, and continue cooking, stirring, until the vegetable extract is well mixed and the water has completely evaporated. Turn off the heat and leave to cool for a few minutes.
3   Spread the oats out on a baking sheet and toast in the oven for 10 minutes. Add to the onions and stir well (if the pan isn't big enough for this, or if it's easier, transfer the onions to a mixing bowl).

4   Use the potato to line the base of the tin, arranging it in concentric circles. Add the cheese, parsley and eggs to the onions and oats, and mix well. Spoon into the tin, on top of the potatoes and level the top with the back of the spoon. Cover the tin with foil.

5   Bake for 30 minutes. Turn out onto a baking sheet and remove the lining paper. Return to the oven for a further 5 minutes to allow the potato topping to brown a little. Cool on the baking sheet for a few minutes, then cut into wedges and serve hot.

FOR EXTRA FIBRE

Serve with an apple and fennel salad (serves 4): trim 250g fennel, halve and remove the central core, then thinly slice lengthways. Quarter, core and thinly slice 1 large eating apple. Put in a bowl with 50g roughly chopped walnuts or pecan nuts. In a small bowl, whisk together 1 tsp maple syrup, 1 tsp Dijon mustard and 1 ½ tsp apple or cider vinegar, with salt and pepper to taste. Whisk in 4 tbsp rapeseed or olive oil and 1 tsp poppy seeds (optional). Drizzle over the salad and toss everything together.

Suitable for vegetarians. Vegans should use a vegan cheese substitute suitable for cooking.

Vegetable Tikka Masala

This colourful and easy vegetarian curry makes a satisfying main course. Vary the vegetables to suit your taste or what's in season. Serve with brown basmati rice or wholewheat naan breads (see recipe under Extra Fibre below).

SERVES 4

1 tbsp rapeseed or sunflower oil
2 red onions, finely sliced
600ml boiling vegetable stock
2–3 tbsp tikka masala curry paste
1 small cauliflower, broken into florets
½ butternut squash, cut into 2cm chunks
2 medium courgettes, halved lengthways and cut into 2cm chunks
400g can chickpeas, drained and rinsed, or 250g cooked chickpeas (page 25)
2 tsp cornflour
100ml natural yogurt
3 tbsp chopped fresh coriander
wholewheat naan bread or brown basmati rice, to serve

1   Heat the oil in a large frying pan. Add the onions and cook over a low heat for 7–8 minutes, stirring frequently until soft. Add a spoonful or two of the stock if they start to stick.

2   Add the curry paste and cook for a further 1 minute, then gradually add the stock, stirring. Add the cauliflower and butternut squash to the pan. Bring to the boil, then reduce the heat, cover the pan with a lid and simmer for 15 minutes.

3   Add the courgettes and chickpeas, and simmer for a further 15 minutes or until all the vegetables are just tender.

4 Blend the cornflour in a small bowl with a few spoonfuls of the yogurt, then stir in the remaining yogurt. Add to the vegetable mixture a third at a time, stirring until blended. Let the curry bubble for a few minutes, then turn off the heat. Stir in the coriander and serve in warmed bowls with wholewheat naan bread or on a bed of brown basmati rice.

FOR EXTRA FIBRE

Serve the curry with wholewheat naan bread: mix 250g wholewheat self-raising flour and 1 tsp salt in a bowl. Add 2 tbsp natural yogurt, then gradually work in 125ml tepid water to make a soft, slightly sticky dough. Knead the dough in the bowl for a few seconds until smooth, then cover the bowl with cling film and leave to rest for 1 hour. Divide the dough into 8 pieces and shape each into an oval. Roll out each on a lightly floured surface to an oval about 20cm long and 1cm thick. Heat 2 tsp ghee or oil in a large non-stick heavy-based frying pan over a medium heat and cook 2 naans at a time for 3–4 minutes on each side until puffy and speckled with brown spots. Serve as soon as possible while still warm and fresh.

Suitable for vegetarians. Vegans should use a plain soya or nut milk or coconut yogurt.

Desserts

Although fresh or tinned fruit in juice makes an excellent and easy fibre-rich dessert, now and then you might want something a little more exciting or elaborate for Sunday lunch, entertaining or a special occasion. There's plenty of choice here, from hot desserts such as quick-and-easy Oaty Apricot Crumble (page 138) and divine Sticky Toffee Puddings (page 140), to chilled delights that you can make the day before, such as No-Bake Blueberry Cheesecake (page 134) and Raspberry and Rose Frozen Yogurt (page 146). This tempting chapter is perfect for anyone with a sweet tooth.

Try old-fashioned favourites given a fibre-rich twist, such as Banana Rice Pudding (page 136); it's made with brown rice and sweetened with dried bananas, so no extra sugar is needed. From the traditional to the more contemporary, and whatever the season, you'll find something here to suit everyone. They all contain a generous amount of fibre and err on the healthy side, so you can eat and enjoy them without feeling in the least bit guilty!

No-Bake Blueberry Cheesecake

As an alternative to the traditional biscuit base, this one is made with crunchy bran flakes, which works well with the citrus and blueberry filling. Some of the blueberries are lightly cooked and folded into the filling, the rest are mixed with syrupy juices for the topping.

SERVES 6-8

450g blueberries
2 tbsp clear apple juice
125g caster sugar
350g mascarpone cheese
zest and juice of 1 lime
juice of 2 lemons
2 tbsp redcurrant jelly

For the base:
50g butter or margarine
2 tbsp clear apple juice
100g bran flakes

1   To make the base, line a 20cm loose-based round shallow cake tin with baking paper. Gently heat the butter and apple juice in a saucepan over a medium heat until melted. Turn off the heat. Put the bran flakes in a plastic bag and lightly crush them with a rolling pin, then stir them into the melted mixture. Transfer to the tin and press down firmly with your fingers. Chill in the fridge while making the filling.

2   Put 150g of the blueberries in a saucepan with the apple juice and 50g of the sugar. Gently cook over a medium heat for 2-3 minutes until the berries just start to burst. Turn off the heat and leave to cool, then remove the berries using a slotted spoon into a small bowl, leaving the juices behind in the pan.

3   Put the remaining 75g sugar in a bowl. Add the mascarpone cheese, lime zest and juice and lemon juice. Beat until smooth and creamy. Add the cooked blueberries and lightly fold into the mixture to create a rippled effect. Spoon and scrape the mixture on top of the bran flake base, levelling the top smooth. Chill in the fridge for an hour.

4   Simmer the reserved blueberry juices in the pan for 2–3 minutes, until slightly reduced and syrupy. Add the redcurrant jelly and gently heat until melted. Turn off the heat and leave to cool for 2–3 minutes. Stir the remaining 200g blueberries into the mixture, leave until just cool, but not setting, then spoon over the top of the cheesecake.

5   Chill the cheesecake for a further 2–3 hours until very firm, or overnight if you prefer. Carefully remove from the tin and serve in wedges.

TIP

The acid in the lime and lemon juice works with the mascarpone cheese to set the cheesecake, so don't worry that the mixture is quite soft when spooning it into the tin.

Suitable for vegetarians.

Banana Rice Pudding

Rice pudding made with brown rice has a slightly nuttier texture than when made with white rice. The dried bananas soften during cooking, flavouring and sweetening the mixture. You can serve with a drizzle of honey or some soft brown sugar, but you will probably find it's sweet enough already.

SERVES 4

1 tsp butter, softened, or coconut oil
50g dried bananas, broken into small pieces
85g brown rice
750ml semi-skimmed milk (see Tip)
a little freshly grated nutmeg or a pinch of ground cinnamon (optional)
honey or soft brown sugar, to serve (optional)

1   Preheat the oven to 150°C/fan oven 130°C/gas 2. Use the butter or coconut oil to grease a 900ml ovenproof dish. Tip the dried banana pieces into the dish.

2   Rinse the rice in a sieve under cold running water. Drain well, then add to the banana pieces. Pour the milk into a small saucepan and gently heat until it reaches boiling point. (Alternatively, heat the milk in a jug in the microwave.) Pour over the bananas and rice, then stir to mix.

3   Bake for 1 hour, then stir the mixture and sprinkle the top with freshly grated nutmeg, if you like. Return to the oven and cook for a further 45–50 minutes until the rice is cooked and most of the milk has been absorbed.

4   Allow the pudding to stand at room temperature for a few minutes, then spoon into bowls and serve drizzled with a little honey, if you like.

TIP

UHT semi-skimmed milk is particularly good for this recipe, as the heat treatment gives it a creamy flavour.

FOR EXTRA FIBRE

Sprinkle some toasted coconut flakes over the top of the rice pudding when serving.

Suitable for vegetarians. Vegans should use a non-dairy milk such as almond or coconut.

Oaty Apricot Crumble

Make this with fresh apricots when in season and abundant. It is subtly flavoured with cardamom, which has a natural affinity with this fruit. Nuts, oats and seeds add a contrasting crunchy texture to the soft and juicy fruit.

SERVES 4

450g fresh apricots, stoned and quartered
1–2 tbsp caster sugar, to taste
50g plain wholemeal or wholewheat flour
50g rolled oats
50g butter or baking margarine, diced
25g light brown sugar
25g hazelnuts, roughly chopped
1 tbsp sunflower seeds
2 green cardamom pods, split open and the seeds finely crushed
custard, to serve

1 Preheat the oven to 190°C/fan oven 170°C/mark 5. Mix the apricots with caster sugar to taste, then put in a 1.2-litre capacity ovenproof dish or divide among 4 individual dishes.

2 Put the flour and oats in a mixing bowl. Add the butter and rub in with your fingertips. Stir in the light brown sugar, hazelnuts, sunflower seeds and crushed cardamom seeds.

3 Sprinkle the topping mixture over the apricots. Bake for 20–25 minutes until the topping is lightly browned and crisp and the fruit is tender. Allow to cool for a few minutes before serving with custard.

Variation

For an apple and ginger crumble, use 6 eating apples, quartered, cored and thinly sliced (no need to peel). Leave out the cardamom seeds and add 1 tsp ground ginger to the topping.

TIP

If you use really ripe and sweet apricots for making this crumble, you might find that you can cut down on the sugar added to the fruit.

FOR EXTRA FIBRE

Add 2 tbsp wheatgerm or 1 tbsp oat bran to the flour and oat mixture when rubbing in the fat.

Suitable for vegetarians. Vegans should use a vegan baking margarine and serve with vegan custard made with non-dairy milk.

Sticky Toffee Puddings

Typically, sticky toffee puddings are high in both fat and sugar. This version doesn't contain the usual butter, but it still has a high sugar content so make sure this dessert is an occasional rather than regular treat. The puddings have a moist texture achieved by steaming in a bain-marie (a shallow container filled with hot water) in the oven.

MAKES 4

butter or oil, for greasing
150ml maple syrup
175g dried stoned dates, chopped
2 tsp vanilla extract
2 eggs, separated
85g self-raising wholemeal flour
a pinch of salt
1 tbsp milk

For the sauce:
100g dried stoned dates, chopped
250ml boiling water
200ml full-fat coconut milk
1 tsp vanilla extract
a pinch of salt

1   To make the sauce, put the 100g dates in a heatproof bowl and pour over the boiling water. Leave to soak for 30 minutes, then strain, reserving both the dates and soaking liquid. Put the dates in a blender with about half the coconut milk, the vanilla extract and salt, and blend until very smooth. Add the remaining coconut milk, blend again, then pour the sauce into a small pan. Leave to one side.

2   Preheat the oven to 180°C/fan oven 160°C/gas 4. Lightly grease and line the bases of four individual 200ml pudding basins with baking paper. Spoon 1 tbsp of the maple syrup into the base of each.

3 To make the puddings, put the 175g dates in a saucepan. Measure the reserved soaking liquid from the sauce and make up to 175ml with boiling water. Pour over the dates. Bring to the boil, then reduce the heat, half-cover the pan with a lid and simmer for 3–4 minutes until the dates are pulpy. Leave to cool for 10 minutes.

4 Tip the date mixture into a blender, add the remaining maple syrup and vanilla extract, and blend to a smooth purée. Pour into a mixing bowl. Beat in the egg yolks one at a time, then sift the flour and salt over the mixture, adding the bran left in the sieve, add the milk and gently mix together.

5 Whisk the egg whites in a clean bowl until stiff enough to hold soft peaks. Fold a third of the egg whites into the mixture to loosen it, then gently fold in the remainder. Spoon into the prepared pudding basins.

6 Cover each pudding basin with a piece of greased foil and put in an ovenproof dish or a small roasting tin. Pour in enough near-boiling water to come halfway up the sides of the basins. Bake for 50 minutes or until a skewer inserted into the centre comes out clean.

7 Heat the date sauce until piping hot. Carefully turn out the puddings onto warmed serving plates and serve with the sauce poured over the top.

FOR EXTRA FIBRE

For date and walnut sponges, fold 50g chopped toasted walnuts into the mixture with the flour.

Suitable for vegetarians.

Cherry Bakewell Sponge

Wholemeal flour is great in many puddings and bakes, but in some such as this almondy sponge, white flour gives the dessert a better flavour and a lighter texture. Here fibre is provided by the fruity cherry base and almond topping instead.

SERVES 4

480g bag frozen pitted dark cherries
6 tbsp cherry jam
1 tbsp water
125g butter, softened
125g caster sugar
2 eggs, lightly beaten
30g self-raising flour, sifted
100g ground almonds
a pinch salt
50g flaked almonds
2 tsp icing sugar, for dusting
custard, to serve

1 If time allows, put the bag of cherries on a plate or in a bowl and leave them in the fridge overnight to defrost or for 2 hours at room temperature. If you don't have time for this, cook the cherries from frozen.
2 Put the cherries in a pan with the jam and water. Gently cook over a low heat, stirring occasionally for 3–4 minutes until the jam has melted. Tip into an ovenproof dish.
3 Preheat the oven to 180°C/fan oven 160°C/gas 4. Put the butter in a bowl and add the sugar, eggs, flour, ground almonds and salt. Beat together with an electric whisk or wooden spoon until light. Carefully spoon on top of the cherries and spread out evenly.

4 Sprinkle the top of the sponge mixture with flaked almonds and bake for 35–40 minutes until a skewer inserted into the sponge layer comes out clean. Cover the top with a piece of foil if the almonds start to brown too much.

5 Remove from the oven and lightly dust the top with icing sugar. Leave to cool for 5 minutes before serving warm with custard.

Variation

For an apple and blackberry base, put 1 peeled, cored and chopped cooking apple in a pan with 350g frozen blackberries (preferably defrosted), 6 tbsp blackberry or redcurrant jelly and 2 tbsp caster sugar. Gently cook for 3–4 minutes, until the jam has melted and the apple is just beginning to soften. Complete the recipe as before.

Suitable for vegetarians.

Pumpkin Pie

This classic American tart is perfect during the autumn months when pumpkins and other squashes are readily available. The pastry case is made with half white and half wholemeal flour, so it is still light and crumbly while adding a little extra fibre to this dessert.

SERVES 6

750g pumpkin or butternut squash, cut into chunks
150g caster sugar
½ tsp freshly grated nutmeg
1 tsp ground cinnamon
a pinch of salt
2 eggs, lightly beaten
25g butter, melted
175ml milk

For the pastry:
75g plain white flour
75g plain wholemeal flour
75g cool butter, cubed
25g icing sugar, sifted
1 egg yolk

1 To make the pastry, sift the flours into a bowl, tipping in the bran left in the sieve. Rub in the butter using your fingertips until the mixture resembles fine breadcrumbs. Stir in the sugar. Mix together the egg yolk and 1 tbsp cold water, add to the dry ingredients and mix to form a soft dough, adding a few more drops of water if needed. Wrap the dough in cling film and chill in the fridge for 30 minutes.

2 Meanwhile, put the pumpkin in a pan and pour in just enough cold water to cover. Bring to the boil, reduce the heat, half-cover the pan with a lid and simmer for 15 minutes or until tender. Drain well and leave until barely warm.

3 Preheat the oven to 200°C/fan oven 180°C/gas 6 and put a baking sheet in to heat. Roll out the pastry and use to line a 23cm shallow, fluted, loose-based tart tin. Prick the base with a fork, line with a sheet of baking paper or foil, and weigh it down with ceramic baking beans or dried beans. Bake for 10 minutes, then lift out the paper or foil and beans and bake for a further 5 minutes.

4 While the pastry case is cooking, push the cooled pumpkin through a sieve into a bowl. Add the sugar, spices and salt, and mix well. Stir in the eggs, followed by the butter and milk.

5 Pour the pumpkin mixture into the pastry case and bake for 10 minutes. Reduce the oven temperature to 180°C/fan oven 160°C/gas 4 and bake for a further 30–35 minutes until the filling has just set. Serve warm or cold.

TIP

Cool the cooked pumpkin in a colander, allowing the steam to escape, so that it is as dry as possible before mashing.

Suitable for vegetarians.

Raspberry and Rose Frozen Yogurt

This pretty pink summery dessert is flavoured with rosewater, which adds a slightly exotic taste without overpowering the fruity raspberries. Sieving the raspberry purée does reduce the fibre content a little but it is essential to give the frozen yogurt a smooth velvety finish.

SERVES 4

250g raspberries, plus extra for serving

2 tbsp raspberry jam

1 tbsp rosewater

1–2 tbsp raspberry liqueur, to taste, such as framboise (optional) (see Tip)

20g icing sugar, sifted

250ml full-fat Greek yogurt

1 Put the raspberries and jam in a saucepan. Heat very gently for about 5 minutes, stirring occasionally until the raspberries are pulpy. Remove from the heat and press the raspberries and their juices through a stainless steel or nylon sieve into a bowl. Discard the pips left in the sieve.

2 Stir in the rosewater and the liqueur, if using. Sift over the icing sugar and stir in, then whisk in the yogurt, a third at a time, until blended.

3 Pour the mixture into an ice-cream maker and freeze according to the manufacturer's instructions. Alternatively, pour the mixture into a freezer-proof container and freeze. Whisk after freezing for 1 hour, then whisk again every 30 minutes for the next 2 hours or until very thick and slushy. Freeze until solid.

4 If storing in the freezer for more than 4 hours, transfer to the fridge about 15 minutes before serving to allow it to soften a little. Scoop into bowls and serve with extra fresh raspberries to decorate.

Variation

For a blackberry frozen yogurt, use blackberries instead of raspberries, blackberry or blackcurrant jam and a blackberry or blackcurrant liqueur such as crème de cassis.

TIP

Don't be tempted to use more than 2 tbsp of liqueur when making this – too much alcohol will prevent the mixture from freezing.

FOR EXTRA FIBRE

Sprinkle the frozen yogurt with toasted flaked almonds or chopped hazelnuts when serving.

Suitable for vegetarians.

Chocolate and Coconut Ice Cream

High-fibre desserts don't have to be based on fresh fruit. This is an indulgent chocolate dessert in which dried dates add a rich texture and sweetness without a noticeable date flavour.

SERVES 4

200g stoned Medjool or soft dates, roughly chopped
60g unsweetened cacao or cocoa powder
2 tsp vanilla extract
200ml milk (full-fat or semi-skimmed)
400g can coconut milk, chilled (see Tip)

1   Put the dates in a food processor with the cacao. Add the vanilla extract and dairy milk. Blend until the mixture is a smooth glossy paste, stopping every 15 seconds to scrape down the sides of the food processor.
2   Add a little of the coconut milk, then continue blending and adding more coconut milk until it is all added to make a smooth, thick mixture.
3   Pour the mixture into an ice-cream maker and freeze according to the manufacturer's instructions. Alternatively, pour the mixture into a freezer-proof container and freeze. Whisk after freezing for 1 hour, then whisk again every 30 minutes for the next two hours or until very thick and slushy. Freeze until solid.
4   Allow the ice cream to soften a little in the fridge 15 minutes before serving. Scoop into bowls and serve straight away.

Variation

You can make a really simple banana ice cream (a great way to use up over-ripe bananas, left in the fruit bowl). Peel and thinly slice 4 very ripe bananas into a freezer-proof container and freeze for 3–4 hours. Tip the frozen bananas into a food processor, add 4 tbsp milk (any kind) and blend to make a smooth ice cream. Spoon into chilled bowls and serve straight away, scattered with dried banana pieces.

> **TIP**
>
> Use full-fat coconut milk for a smooth, creamy ice cream or half-fat coconut milk if you want a less rich, lower-calorie version. Chilling the can in the fridge overnight or popping it in the freezer 30 minutes before making will help the ice cream freeze faster.
>
> Suitable for vegetarians. To make a vegan version use almond, hazelnut or coconut drinking milk instead of dairy milk.

Peaches and Cream Winter Fool

Fresh peaches have a very short season, but you can still enjoy their flavour throughout the year by using dried fruit. In this creamy dessert yogurt is combined with whipping cream to make a rich-tasting fool that isn't overly high in fat or calories.

SERVES 4
300g ready-to-eat dried peaches
2 tbsp peach schnapps, orange liqueur or orange juice
200ml orange juice
5 tbsp medium oatmeal
1 tbsp clear honey (see Tip)
150ml whipping cream
150ml natural low-fat yogurt

1 Snip 50g of the dried peaches into small pieces using kitchen scissors. Put in a small bowl and spoon over the schnapps. Leave to soak.

2 Cut the remaining peaches into quarters and put in a small heavy-based saucepan. Pour over the orange juice and leave to soak for a few minutes.

3 Meanwhile, line the rack in the grill pan with foil and preheat the grill to high. Spread the oatmeal over the foil and toast under the grill for 3 minutes or until the oatmeal is golden, stirring once or twice. Leave to one side to cool.

4 Bring the peaches in the pan to the boil, then reduce the heat, cover the pan with a lid and simmer gently for 10 minutes or until the fruit is very tender. Cool a little, then purée with the honey in a food processor until smooth.

5 Whip the cream in a mixing bowl until thick. Add the yogurt and whip to mix with the cream. Fold in 4 tbsp of the oatmeal.

6 Layer alternate spoonfuls of the peach purée and cream mixture into 4 glasses or glass bowls, then swirl the mixture slightly using a spoon or skewer to give a marbled effect. Spoon the marinated fruits on top and sprinkle with the remaining 1 tbsp oatmeal just before serving.

Variation

Dried apricots or dried prunes can be used instead of the peaches, if you prefer.

TIP

If you use a mild bio yogurt rather than a sharper natural yogurt, you probably won't need to add the honey to the peach purée.

Suitable for vegetarians.

Pineapple and Orange Jelly

Homemade fruit jelly is a real treat, a million miles away from some packet jellies containing artificial colours and flavours. Canned fruit contains as much fibre as the fresh variety, and a few cans of fruit in juice is a useful larder standby.

SERVES 4

220g can pineapple chunks in juice

about 450ml pure orange or pineapple juice, or a mixture of
the two

4 tsp powdered gelatine

3 oranges

1   Drain the pineapple, reserving the juice. Divide the chunks among 4 individual serving glasses or glass bowls and put in the fridge to chill the glasses. Measure the juice and make up to 600ml with the orange juice.

2   Spoon 4 tbsp of the fruit juice into a small heatproof bowl. Sprinkle the gelatine over and leave to soak for 5 minutes. Put the bowl over a pan of near-boiling water and leave for 2–3 minutes, then stir until the gelatine has completely dissolved.

3   Cool the gelatine for 4–5 minutes, then add to the remaining fruit juice and stir well. Pour a little jelly over the pineapple pieces to just cover them and return the glasses to the fridge for 30 minutes or until the jelly is starting to set. Leave the remaining jelly at room temperature.

4 Using a sharp knife, cut a thin slice of peel and pith from each end of an orange. Put cut-side down on a plate and cut off the peel and pith in strips. Remove any remaining pith. Cut out each segment leaving the membrane behind. Squeeze the remaining juice from the membrane and add to the jelly mixture. Repeat for the remaining oranges. Divide the orange segments between the glasses. Pour the remaining jelly into the glasses. Chill in the fridge for at least 2 hours or until completely set.

Variation

You can use other fruits in this jelly such as sliced mango, or seedless green or black grapes (small children can choke on whole grapes, so cut them in half if serving to children). Don't use fresh pineapple, though, as it contains an enzyme that prevents jelly from setting; the heat treatment in canning destroys this enzyme.

TIP

Chilling the glasses of jelly before adding the orange segments will allow it to set in two layers of fruit, otherwise all the fruit will sink to the bottom.

Fresh Fig Compote

Fresh figs have a unique taste and a soft texture that contrasts with their slightly crunchy edible seeds. They are high in minerals including potassium, calcium and iron as well as being an excellent source of soluble fibre. Fresh figs don't keep for long, so if you grow your own and have a glut, this is the perfect dessert to make.

SERVES 4

350ml clear unsweetened apple juice or white grape juice
1 vanilla pod
6 tbsp clear honey
12 slightly under-ripe fresh figs
1 tsp lemon juice
Greek-style yogurt, to serve (optional)

1   Pour the apple juice into a frying pan just large enough to hold the figs (which will be halved) in a single layer.
2   Split the vanilla pod in half lengthways and scrape the black seeds into the pan. Add the vanilla pod and honey, then bring the mixture to a gentle simmer.
3   Meanwhile, wash the figs and pierce the skins several times with a fine skewer or sharp knife (this will let the flavours penetrate the fruit). Cut in half lengthways through the stem to the base, then carefully add to the pan, cut side up.
4   Cover the pan with a lid and simmer for 5–6 minutes, basting the cut sides of the figs occasionally with the cooking juices. Remove the figs from the pan with a slotted spoon and transfer to a serving dish.
5   Bring the syrup to a rapid boil and cook uncovered until slightly thickened and reduced to about 200ml. Leave to cool, then stir in the lemon juice.

6 Strain the syrup over the figs (use a fine sieve if you want to remove the vanilla seeds). Allow to stand at room temperature for 1 hour before serving, or cover and chill in the fridge for up to 48 hours. Serve with Greek-style yogurt, if you like.

TIP

Rinse and dry the vanilla pod; it can be re-used several times.

Suitable for vegetarians. Vegans should serve with non-dairy yogurt.

Chocolate and Avocado Mousse

Using avocado in a chocolate mousse has been a trendy dish on the vegan scene for the last few years. Avocados are surprisingly high in fibre, so if you haven't tried this dessert before, give it a go. It's absolutely delicious and the flavour of avocado is barely noticeable – they give the mousse a rich, creamy texture without the need for eggs or dairy.

SERVES 4

75g dark chocolate with a high cocoa content (at least 70 per cent), broken into squares

2 tbsp maple syrup

2 large ripe avocados

2 tbsp cacao or unsweetened cocoa powder, sieved, plus extra for serving

4 tbsp almond milk or coconut milk drink (or semi-skimmed milk if non-vegan)

2 tsp vanilla extract

a small pinch of salt (optional)

1   Put the chocolate in a small heatproof bowl over a pan of very hot (not boiling) water. Leave for 2–3 minutes, then stir until melted. Remove the bowl from the heat. Stir in the maple syrup.

2   Meanwhile, halve the avocados and remove the stones. Peel, then roughly chop the flesh and put in a food processor with the cacao, milk, vanilla extract and salt, if using. Blend to a smooth purée.

3   Scrape down the sides of the food processor, add the melted chocolate mixture and blend again until smooth.

4   Divide the mixture between four individual glasses or ramekins and chill in the fridge for at least 2 hours before serving. Sprinkle over a light dusting of cacao, if you like.

NUTRITIONAL NOTE

Avocados are a great source of vitamin E and contain iron, potassium and niacin. Although high in fat (and therefore calories), most of it is the beneficial monounsaturated type, currently believed to protect against heart disease and to lower blood pressure.

Suitable for vegetarians and vegans if made with a chocolate that has no dairy content.

Baking

From deliciously textured breads and moist rolls, to light-as-air scones, sticky cakes and crumbly cookies, you'll find all manner of baked goods in this chapter.

Although you can buy fibre-rich breads, there's truly nothing quite like the aroma and flavour of freshly baked homemade bread. Here, you'll discover Sweet Potato Bread Rolls (page 160) and a Multi-Grain Loaf (page 162), which includes unsweetened muesli as well as rye and wholemeal flours to give it a fantastic taste and texture. A Sun-Dried Tomato and Olive Focaccia (page 164) is perfect for picnics, to serve at barbecues or to accompany simple grilled foods and salads.

When you are looking for a little something to enjoy mid-morning or mid-afternoon, don't resort to unhealthy deep-fried doughnuts or white pastries layered with cream. This is the perfect time to add extra fibre to your day with a small slice of Carrot and Coconut Cake (page 174) or a couple of Oat and Apple or Wholemeal Spelt and Honey Cookies. For those who need to follow a gluten-free diet, or have friends who can't eat gluten, there are a couple of cakes to suit them, too, which everyone will enjoy: Banana and Date Loaf (page 170) and Chocolate Chunk Black-Bean Brownies (page 176).

Not everyone has a sweet tooth, of course, and for those who prefer savouries, bake some Cheddar and Watercress Scones (page 168) or Cheese and Seed Oatcakes (page 186).

Sweet Potato Bread Rolls

These soft light-textured rolls are a great compromise for those who feel that wholemeal bread is healthier but prefer the taste and texture of white. Sweet potatoes are rich in dietary fibre, and eating just one of these rolls will provide you with around 1.7g fibre.

MAKES 12 ROLLS

225g orange-fleshed sweet potatoes
1½ tsp salt
2 tsp sunflower or rapeseed oil, plus extra for greasing
150ml skimmed milk, plus 1 tbsp
450g strong white bread flour, plus extra for dusting
7g sachet (2 tsp) easy-blend dried yeast
2 eggs, beaten
oil, for greasing
2 tbsp poppy or sesame seeds, for sprinkling

1   Thinly peel the sweet potatoes and cut into large chunks. Cook in a saucepan of boiling water for 12 minutes or until tender. Drain well in a colander, then mash with the salt and oil until very smooth. Stir in the 150ml milk. Leave the mixture to cool until lukewarm.

2   Meanwhile, line a baking sheet with baking paper. Sift the flour into a large bowl, stir in the yeast and make a hollow in the centre.

3   Reserve 1 tbsp of the beaten eggs. Add the sweet potato mixture and remaining beaten eggs to the flour and mix to a soft dough. Turn out onto a lightly floured work surface and knead the dough for 10 minutes or until smooth and elastic.

4   Put the dough in a lightly oiled bowl, cover with cling film or a tea towel and leave in a warm place for 1 hour or until the dough has doubled in size.

5 Turn out the dough and knock it back with your knuckles to deflate it, then divide it into 12 pieces and shape each into a round roll. Arrange on the prepared baking sheet, cover with oiled cling film and leave for 20 minutes or until well risen. Towards the end of the rising time, preheat the oven to 200°C/fan oven 180°C/gas 6.

6 Carefully remove the cling film. Mix the reserved beaten egg with the 1 tbsp milk and use to brush the tops of the rolls, then generously sprinkle with seeds. Bake for 12 minutes or until risen and golden brown. Lift onto a wire rack, cover with a clean tea towel to keep the rolls soft and leave them to cool.

TIP

These rolls are a lovely pale orange colour. If you want whiter bread rolls, choose sweet potatoes with a creamy-white flesh instead of ones with an orange flesh.

NUTRITIONAL NOTE

As well as fibre, starchy sweet potatoes are rich in numerous minerals including iron, calcium and selenium, plus most of the B-group vitamins, vitamin C and the antioxidant beta-carotene, which the body converts to vitamin A.

Suitable for vegetarians

Multi-Grain Bread

No-added-sugar muesli is a great fibre-rich addition to this loaf, which also contains rye flour, wholemeal flour and wheatgerm. Packed with nutrients, it's delicious served fresh with a little spread or butter and is also good toasted.

MAKES 1 LOAF (ABOUT 8 SLICES)
1 tsp clear honey
150ml skimmed milk, warmed
100g no-added-sugar muesli
200g strong white bread flour, plus extra for dusting
100g rye flour
75g wholemeal bread flour
1 tsp salt
25g wheatgerm
1 tsp easy-blend dried yeast
300ml warm water
oil, for greasing
beaten egg or milk, for glazing
15g sunflower or pumpkin seeds or 1 tbsp poppy seeds, for sprinkling

1   Stir the honey into the warm milk. Put the muesli in a bowl and pour over the milk. Leave to soak for 15 minutes. Meanwhile, sift the flours and salt into a large mixing bowl, adding the bran and any grains left in the sieve. Stir in the wheatgerm and yeast.

2   Make a well in the centre, then add the soaked muesli and about 250ml of the warm water. Mix together to form a soft dough, adding more water if needed (the amount will depend on the muesli used, so you might not need it all).

3   Turn out the dough onto a lightly floured work surface and knead for 5 minutes or until smooth. Put in a lightly oiled bowl, cover with cling film and leave to rise for 1 ½ hours or until doubled in size.

4 Knock back the dough with your knuckles to deflate it, then shape it into an oval about 25cm long. Using a sharp knife, make several diagonal cuts across the top of the loaf. Carefully transfer it to a baking sheet lined with baking paper, cover loosely with oiled cling film and leave to rise for 20–30 minutes until well risen.

5 Preheat the oven to 200°C/fan oven 180°C/gas 6. Carefully remove the cling film from the loaf. Brush the top with beaten egg and sprinkle with seeds.

6 Bake for 40–45 minutes until firm and well browned and the bread sounds hollow when the underneath is tapped. Cool on a wire rack, covered with a tea towel to stop the crust from becoming too hard.

TIP

For a lighter textured loaf, use white rye flour instead of rye flour. Although not as rich in fibre as classic rye flour, this still has a good content and contains 5g fibre per 100g of flour.

Suitable for vegetarians. Also suitable for vegans if non-dairy milk is used and maple syrup is used instead of honey (also check that your chosen muesli is for vegans, as some contain added milk powder).

Sun-Dried Tomato and Olive Focaccia

This olive-oil flatbread from the northern shores of the Mediterranean is traditionally made with white flour but is equally good made with a mixture of wholemeal and white. The olives and sun-dried tomatoes add both fibre and a rich flavour to the bread.

MAKES 1 LOAF

4 tbsp olive oil, plus extra for greasing
300g strong wholemeal bread flour
200g strong white bread flour, plus extra for dusting
1½ tsp salt
2 tbsp wheatgerm
12 pitted green olives, halved
8 sun-dried tomatoes, chopped
1½ tsp easy-blend dried yeast
400–425ml lukewarm water
a few fresh rosemary sprigs (optional), divided into small
   sprigs

1 Line a 25 × 35cm shallow tin with baking paper, then lightly grease the base and sides of with olive oil.
2 Sift the flours and salt into a large bowl, adding the bran left in the sieve, then stir in the wheatgerm, olives and tomatoes. Sprinkle the yeast over the top of the flour, then make a hollow in the centre of the dry ingredients. Add 2 tbsp of the oil and 400ml of the lukewarm water and mix to a soft dough, adding a little more water if needed.
3 Turn out onto a lightly floured work surface and knead for 10 minutes or until smooth and elastic. Put the dough in a clean bowl, cover with cling film or a tea towel and leave to rise in a warm place for 1 hour or until doubled in size.

4   Turn out the risen dough and knock it back with your knuckles to deflate it. Roll out the dough into a rectangle, put it in the prepared tin, then push the dough to the edges with your fingertips. Loosely cover with oiled cling film and leave in a warm place for 30 minutes or until well risen.

5   Preheat the oven to 200°C/fan oven 180°C/gas 6. Using the end of a wooden spoon dipped in flour, make deep dimples all over the dough. Brush the top with the remaining 2 tbsp olive oil. Poke the rosemary, if using, into the holes. Re-cover the focaccia with the cling film and leave to rise for a further 5 minutes.

6   If you have a water spray, spray the top of the loaf with water, or wet your fingers with water and flick the water over the surface (this will help to keep the crust soft). Bake for 20–25 minutes until firm and lightly browned. Transfer to a wire rack and leave to cool for 10 minutes, then carefully remove from the tin and serve warm.

TIP

The tin is an easy way to keep the focaccia in a perfect shape, making it easy to cut into squares or rectangles for serving. If you don't have a tin, roll the dough into a 25cm round and cook it on a baking sheet lined with baking paper. Serve cut into wedges.

Suitable for vegetarians and vegans.

Butternut Squash Cornbread

The vibrant orange flesh of butternut squash and yellow polenta (cornmeal) gives this cornbread a stunning golden colour. It's made with buttermilk (see page 35), which counteracts the sweetness of the squash and ensures an even rise and a light texture. It's excellent served with thick soups and stews.

MAKES 8 WEDGES

40g coconut oil, butter or margarine, plus extra for greasing
2 tbsp clear honey
200g butternut squash, coarsely grated
125g fine yellow polenta (cornmeal)
125g plain flour
1½ tsp baking powder
½ tsp bicarbonate of soda
½ tsp salt
200ml buttermilk (see Tips)
1 egg, lightly beaten

1   Preheat the oven to 200°C/fan oven 180°C/gas 6. Line a 23cm round, shallow cake tin with baking paper and lightly grease. Put the coconut oil and honey in a heavy-based saucepan. Add the butternut squash. Gently heat for a few minutes until the fat has melted. When the mixture is just lukewarm, turn off the heat and stir well.

2   While the butternut squash is warming, put the polenta in a large mixing bowl. Sift over the flour, baking powder, bicarbonate of soda and salt, then stir to combine the dry ingredients. Make a hollow in the centre.

3   Stir the buttermilk into the butternut squash mixture, then stir in the beaten egg. Add to the dry ingredients and mix everything together thoroughly to make a thick batter. Tip and scrape the mixture into the prepared tin and spread evenly.

4 Bake for 20–25 minutes until slightly risen, golden brown and a skewer inserted into the centre comes out clean. Leave to cool in the tin for 10 minutes, then turn out onto a wire rack. Serve cold or warm, cut into 8 wedges.

FOR EXTRA FIBRE

Make the cornbread with plain wholemeal instead of white flour, adding an extra 1 tbsp buttermilk or milk.

TIPS

- Cornbread is best eaten on the same day it is made, but if that's not possible, it can be frozen for up to a month. Allow it to defrost, then gently warm for a few minutes in a low oven before serving.
- If you prefer, use half natural yogurt and half semi-skimmed milk instead of the buttermilk.

Suitable for vegetarians.

Cheddar and Watercress Scones

Packed with flavour, these tasty scones have plenty of fibre but are not heavy like some wholemeal scones, as they are lightened with white self-raising flour as well. They make a great accompaniment to soups, can be added to packed lunches and are lovely as a savoury option at an afternoon tea.

MAKES 8

150g self-raising wholemeal flour
150g self-raising white flour, plus extra for dusting
1 tsp baking powder
50g butter, cut into small cubes
50g rolled (porridge) oats
75g watercress leaves (larger tough stalks removed), chopped
75g mature Cheddar cheese, coarsely grated
120ml semi-skimmed milk, plus extra to glaze
salt and freshly ground black pepper

1 Preheat the oven to 220°C/fan oven 200°C/gas 7. Sift the flours and baking powder into a mixing bowl, adding the bran left in the sieve. Rub the butter into the flour using your fingertips until the mixture resembles fine breadcrumbs.
2 Add the oats, watercress and Cheddar to the bowl, season with salt and pepper and stir to mix evenly. Drizzle the milk over the top and stir with a fork to mix to a dough.
3 Using your hands, pat the dough together into a ball, then knead lightly for just a few seconds on a floured surface. Roll or pat out the dough until it is 2cm thick. Using a 7.5cm plain or fluted cutter, stamp the dough into rounds. Press the trimmings together, re-roll and cut out more scones.
4 Put the scones on a heavy non-stick baking sheet, spacing them slightly apart to allow them space to spread a little and to rise. Lightly brush the tops with milk.

5 Bake for 12–15 minutes until well risen and golden brown (check the bases have browned, too). Remove from the oven and transfer to a wire rack. Cover with a clean tea towel while they are cooling to keep them soft. Eat on the day of making if possible or store in an airtight container for the following day.

TIP

If you want to freeze the scones, do so as soon as they are cool.

FOR EXTRA FIBRE

Add a small amount of toasted pine nuts or seeds such as sunflower or pumpkin seeds to the mixture and sprinkle the glazed tops with a few sesame or poppy seeds before baking.

Suitable for vegetarians.

Banana and Date Loaf

Many cakes are loaded with fat, sugar and starchy white flour. This spicy loaf has minimal fat and is sweetened with bananas and just a little maple syrup. It contains ground flax seeds, almonds and dates instead of flour, which keep the cake lovely and moist. These ingredients also make it suitable for those on a gluten-free diet.

MAKES 1 LOAF (ABOUT 10 SLICES)

30g butter, softened, plus extra for greasing
3 tbsp maple syrup or honey
3 very ripe bananas, weighing about 300g in total (see Tip)
1 tsp ground cinnamon
½ tsp ground ginger
a pinch of salt
3 eggs, lightly beaten
1 tbsp lemon juice
75g stoned dates, chopped
225g ground almonds
30g ground flax seeds (linseed)
½ tsp bicarbonate of soda

1   Lightly grease and line the base and sides of a 900g loaf tin with baking paper. Preheat the oven to 180°C/fan oven 160°C/gas 4. Put the butter and maple syrup in a large bowl and mix together until blended. Peel and mash the bananas until fairly smooth and stir into the butter mixture with the cinnamon, ginger and salt.

2   Gradually beat in the eggs, followed by the lemon juice and dates. Add the ground almonds and flax seeds. Sprinkle the bicarbonate of soda over the top and, working quickly, mix everything together until combined. Scrape and fold the mixture into the prepared tin.

3 Bake for 30 minutes, then very carefully cover the top with a piece of lightly oiled foil to prevent the cake from over-browning. Reduce the oven temperature to 170°C/fan oven 150°C/gas 3 and bake for a further 30–40 minutes until a fine skewer inserted into the centre of the cake comes out clean.

4 Remove from the oven and leave to cool in the tin for 10 minutes, then remove and put on a wire rack to cool completely. Wrap and store the cake in an airtight container for up to 2 days at room temperature or in the fridge for up to a week.

TIP

It's important that the bananas are really ripe for this recipe; the yellow skins should be at least half-covered in dark brown patches and feel quite soft when gently squeezed.

FOR EXTRA FIBRE

Stir 75g lightly toasted chopped walnuts, pecan nuts or almonds into the mix when adding the dates.

Suitable for vegetarians.

Tropical Fruit Malt Teabread

This quick and simple-to-make cake is made using bran cereal, which contains barley malt extract. It has a lovely moist texture and slices beautifully – few will guess that it's based on a breakfast cereal.

MAKES 8-10 SLICES

100g bran cereal, such as All-Bran
275g dried tropical fruit mix, such as dried pineapple, papaya and mango, chopped (see Tip)
300ml semi-skimmed milk
75g soft light brown sugar
100g self-raising flour
1 tsp ground ginger
½ tsp baking powder
butter or spread, to serve (optional)

1   Put the bran cereal in a bowl and add the fruit. Pour over the milk, cover the bowl with cling film and leave to soak at room temperature for 1 hour, or for several hours or overnight in the fridge, if you prefer.

2   Preheat the oven to 180°C/fan oven 160°C/gas mark 4. Lightly grease a 23cm square tin and line with baking paper. Stir the sugar into the soaked bran and fruit mixture. Sift over the flour, ginger and baking powder. Gently fold in but do not over-mix. Spoon and scrape the mixture into the prepared cake tin.

3   Bake the cake for 45–50 minutes until risen and firm. If the top starts to over-brown, cover it with a piece of foil about 30 minutes into the cooking time.

4   Leave the cake to cool in the tin for 10 minutes, then turn out and put on a wire rack to cool completely. Serve thickly sliced, spread with a little butter, if you like.

TIP

If you use a brand of tropical fruit with added sugar, reduce the amount of soft light brown sugar to 50g.

VARIATION

For a mixed fruit cake, use mixed dried fruit (raisins, sultanas and currants) instead of dried tropical fruit and add 1 tsp ground cinnamon or mixed spice instead of ginger.

Suitable for vegetarians. Vegans should use a non-dairy milk such as coconut or almond instead of dairy milk.

Carrot and Coconut Cake

Carrots have been used in British cakes since the Middle Ages. They enjoyed a revival during the Second World War due to sugar rationing and made a popular 'alternative' wedding cake in the 1970s. Carrot cake is still enjoyed as a fashionable coffee-shop slice, where it is usually served with a generous cream cheese frosting. Made here with healthy oil, fibre-rich coconut and toasted hazelnuts add texture and flavour to this version.

CUTS INTO 12 SLICES

100g raisins
zest and 3 tbsp juice of 1 orange
175ml rapeseed or sunflower oil, plus extra for greasing
175g light muscovado sugar
3 eggs, lightly beaten
100g wholemeal self-raising flour
100g white self-raising flour
1 tsp bicarbonate of soda
2 tsp ground cinnamon
½ tsp ground ginger
¼ tsp salt (optional)
275g finely grated carrot (2–3 large carrots)
100g toasted hazelnuts (see Tip page 29)
75g desiccated coconut
1 tsp icing sugar

1 Put the raisins in a bowl and add the orange zest and juice. Leave to one side to soak. Preheat the oven to 160°C/fan oven 140°C/gas 3. Grease and line the base of a deep 23cm round tin or a 20cm square tin with baking paper.

2 Put the sugar in a mixing bowl and break up any lumps by rubbing it between your fingers. Add the oil, then, using an electric hand-mixer, beat on a low speed until well mixed. Gradually add the eggs, beating well after each addition; the mixture will now be thick and creamy.

3 Sift the flours, bicarbonate of soda, cinnamon, ginger and salt, if using, over the mixture, adding the bran left in the sieve. Start to fold in with a metal spoon. When half-combined, add the carrots, hazelnuts, coconut and the soaked raisins, orange rind and juice. Continue folding in until mixed.

4 Tip and scrape the mixture into the prepared tin and level the surface. Bake for 50 minutes–1 hour until risen and firm on top and until a fine skewer comes out clean when inserted into the centre. If the top of the cake starts to over-brown during cooking, cover with a piece of foil.

5 Let the cake cool in the tin for 10 minutes, then turn it out onto a wire rack and leave it to cool completely. When cold, wrap the cake in foil or store in a cake tin or airtight container; it improves if left for a day before slicing and eating. Serve with a light dusting of icing sugar.

TIP

For a cream cheese frosting, beat 50g softened unsalted butter and 50g sifted icing sugar together until creamy. Then beat in 100g full-fat soft cheese at room temperature, the finely grated zest of ½ orange and 1 tsp lemon juice. Spread and swirl over the cooled cake. Sprinkle with some coarsely chopped toasted hazelnuts and desiccated coconut if you like.

Suitable for vegetarians.

Chocolate Chunk Black-Bean Brownies

In the vegan world, black-bean brownies are a well-known and popular bake. Rich, dark and chocolatey, this version is every bit as good as the most decadent high-fat and sugary brownie, but it is much healthier and higher in fibre. The black beans are blended to a thick, floury purée but no one will notice that they are there unless you tell them.

MAKES 9 SQUARES

400g can black beans, drained and rinsed, or 250g cooked black beans (see page 25)

2 tbsp soft light brown sugar

2 tsp vanilla extract

a pinch of salt

30g porridge (rolled) oats

3 tbsp cocoa powder

1 tbsp ground flax seeds (linseed)

75g clear honey or agave syrup

40g coconut oil or cocoa butter, melted

½ tsp baking powder

75g dark chocolate, roughly chopped

1 Grease an 18cm square cake tin and line with baking paper. Preheat the oven to 170°C/fan oven 150°C/gas 3. Put the beans, sugar, vanilla and salt in a food processor and blend for a few seconds until the beans are finely chopped. Scrape down the sides with a spatula.

2 Add the oats, cocoa powder, flax seeds, honey and coconut oil, then sprinkle over the baking powder. Blend again for 2–3 minutes until the mixture is fairly smooth.

3 Add the chopped chocolate and blend for 10–15 seconds until the chocolate is mixed in but still chunky.

4 Spoon and scrape the mixture into the prepared tin and bake for 20–22 minutes until lightly set (the top should be firm and dry but the centre still slightly soft).

5 Leave the brownies to cool in the tin, then mark into squares. Chill in the fridge for several hours to firm them up before carefully removing from the tin and cut into squares. Store in an airtight container in the fridge for up to a week.

TIP

These brownies have a slightly fragile texture, so they are best served on plates.

NUTRITIONAL NOTE

Dark chocolate is high in antioxidants and flavanols (naturally occurring protective compounds that have many benefits including helping to lower blood pressure) and is also naturally high in iron, copper and manganese. Although high in fat, eaten in small quantities it can contribute to a healthy diet.

Suitable for vegetarians and vegans (using agave syrup for vegans).

Oat and Apple Cookies

Apple purée is used in these quick-and-easy cookies to replace some of the fat. It gives them a lovely soft texture as well as a delicious flavour. They will keep for up to a week, stored in an airtight container.

MAKES 14

50g butter, softened, or margarine
100g soft light brown sugar
1 egg yolk
150ml unsweetened apple purée (see Tip)
75g porridge (rolled) oats
175g plain wholemeal flour
½ tsp ground cinnamon
½ tsp bicarbonate of soda
1 tsp icing sugar (optional)

1 Preheat the oven to 190°C/fan oven 170°C/gas 5. Line two baking sheets with baking paper. Put the butter and sugar in a bowl and beat together until blended and creamy.

2 Add the egg yolk and beat into the mixture, followed by the apple purée. Stir in the oats and leave the mixture to stand for 2–3 minutes so that the oats start to absorb some of the moisture.

3 Sift the flour, cinnamon and bicarbonate of soda over the mixture, then tip in the bran left in the sieve. Stir everything together to make a soft dough.

4 With lightly floured hands, shape the mixture into 14 balls, each slightly larger than a walnut. Put them on the prepared baking sheets, spacing them apart to allow the mixture to spread, then flatten each ball slightly (this will stop them from rolling off the baking sheets).

5 Bake for 14–15 minutes until the cookies are lightly browned. Leave them to cool on the baking sheets for 3–4 minutes, then transfer them to a wire rack and leave to cool completely. If you like, dust them with a little icing sugar while they are still warm. Store in an airtight container for up to a week.

TIP

To make apple purée, quarter, core, peel and roughly chop 2 sweet eating apples. Put in a heavy-based saucepan with 2 tbsp water or apple juice. Cook over a low heat for 8–10 minutes until very tender, then mash until smooth, or purée in a food processor. Alternatively, buy a jar of ready-made apple sauce or a sachet of apple purée from the baby-food aisle.

VARIATION

For raisin and coconut cookies, soak 50g raisins in 2 tbsp orange juice for 20 minutes before you start making the cookie dough. Add the soaked raisin mixture and 15g desiccated coconut when stirring in the oats in step 2.

Suitable for vegetarians.

Peanut Butter Cookies

These protein-packed bakes are delicious as a mid-morning snack or occasional treat. They are rolled in crushed bran flakes before baking which gives them a crunchy coating and a fibre boost.

MAKES ABOUT 16

175g crunchy peanut butter (see Tip)
50g butter, at room temperature
50g caster sugar or golden caster sugar
40g light brown sugar
1 egg, lightly beaten
125g self-raising wholemeal flour
1 teaspoon milk
50g bran flakes

1 Preheat the oven to 180°C/fan oven 160°C/gas 4. Line two baking sheets with baking paper. Put the peanut butter and butter in a bowl and beat until blended. Add the sugars and beat again until the mixture is lighter in colour and creamy.

2 Gradually add the egg, beating well after each addition. Sift over the flour, adding the bran left in the sieve. Add the milk, then stir everything together to make a stiff dough.

3 Put the bran flakes on a plate and lightly crush them into slightly smaller pieces. Shape the mixture into balls, slightly bigger than a walnut, then roll in the bran flakes to coat them all over.

4 Put the cookies on the prepared sheets, spacing them apart to allow the mixture to spread, then flatten each ball slightly (this will stop them from rolling off the baking sheets).

5 Bake for 10–12 minutes until firm, then remove them from the oven. Allow the cookies to cool on the baking sheets for 3–4 minutes, then transfer to a wire rack and leave to cool completely. Store in an airtight container for up to a week.

Choose a peanut butter with no added sugar and preferably one made without palm oil. If you have a powerful food processor, it is easy to make your own. Put 175g unsalted roasted peanuts in a food processor and blend until finely chopped. Drizzle 1 tbsp groundnut or sunflower oil over the top and blend until the mixture comes together in a clumpy paste. Stop and scrape down the sides of the food processor and continue processing for 2–3 minutes. At first the peanut butter will get thicker, but it should gradually become creamier. Take care not to overheat your machine – stop for a few minutes if necessary, then process again.

Suitable for vegetarians.

Wholemeal Spelt and Honey Biscuits

Spelt is an ancient grain related to wheat and has a lovely nutty texture. It still contains gluten so it is unsuitable for those with coeliac disease, but some who have a slight intolerance to wheat can tolerate spelt. These little biscuits are really quick and easy to make.

MAKES 20

125g wholemeal spelt flour
1 tsp ground ginger or ground cinnamon
½ tsp baking powder
a pinch salt
3 tbsp rapeseed or sunflower oil
75g clear honey
20 pecan or walnut halves or whole blanched almonds
1 tsp icing sugar
¼ tsp ground cinnamon

1   Preheat the oven to 190°C/fan oven 170°C/gas 5. Line a large baking sheet with baking paper. Sift the flour, ginger, baking powder and salt into a bowl and stir together to mix. Put the oil in a small bowl and add the honey, then stir together. Drizzle over the dry ingredients and mix to a soft dough.

2   Divide the dough into 20 pieces and roll each into a ball. Arrange on the prepared baking sheet, spacing them slightly apart to allow room for them to spread. Top each biscuit with a nut, pressing down lightly while doing this to flatten the cookies very slightly.

3   Bake for 10–12 minutes until slightly darker in colour. Leave to cool on the baking sheet for 2–3 minutes, then transfer to a wire rack.

4 Mix the icing sugar and cinnamon together in a small bowl and lightly dust the tops of the cookies while they are still warm. Leave to cool completely. When cold, store the biscuits in a tin or airtight container for up to 2 weeks.

VARIATION

Instead of whole nuts, scatter the tops with 25g chopped walnuts or pine nuts, pressing them down lightly. Make a filling by creaming together 50g butter, 100g sifted icing sugar and 1 tbsp clear honey, and use to sandwich the biscuits together in pairs.

Suitable for vegetarians. Vegans should use agave syrup, carob syrup or maple syrup instead of honey.

Digestive Biscuits

Slightly sweet and salty, a classic digestive is also the ultimate high-fibre biscuit. This homemade version contains wholemeal flour, oatmeal and oat bran. The biscuits are sliced from a long roll of dough, which you can make ahead and keep in the freezer so that you are ready to bake the biscuits whenever you want to.

MAKES 12 BISCUITS

75g plain wholemeal flour
1/2 tsp baking powder
1/4 tsp bicarbonate of soda
1/4 tsp salt
15g medium oatmeal
10g oat bran
25g unsalted butter, cut into small cubes
50g dark soft brown sugar
2 tbsp milk

1   Sift the flour, baking powder, bicarbonate of soda and salt into a mixing bowl, adding the bran left in the sieve. Stir in the oatmeal and oat bran. Add the butter and rub into the dry ingredients with your fingertips until the mixture resembles fine breadcrumbs.
2   Stir in the sugar, then sprinkle the milk over the top. Stir together to make a soft dough. Turn out the dough onto a piece of baking paper and shape into a log about 12cm long. Roll the dough backwards and forwards a few times to make a smooth cylinder. Twist the ends of the baking paper to seal. Chill in the fridge for 30 minutes or freeze for another day, if you prefer.
3   If you have frozen the dough, remove from the freezer and leave in the fridge for at least 1 hour to defrost. Preheat the oven to 190°C/fan oven 170°C/gas 5. Unwrap the dough and use the baking paper to line a baking sheet.

4 Using a sharp knife, cut the roll of dough across into slices about 8mm thick. Roll the log of dough a little each time you slice so that the biscuits stay round.

5 Put the biscuits on the prepared baking sheet and prick them in several places with a fork. Bake for 10–12 minutes until lightly browned.

6 Leave the biscuits on the baking sheet for 2–3 minutes to firm up, then transfer to a wire rack to cool completely. Store them in an airtight tin for up to a week.

FOR EXTRA FIBRE

Lightly toast 1 tbsp sesame seeds in a dry non-stick frying pan for 3–4 minutes over a low heat, stirring frequently until golden. Tip onto a plate to cool and stir them into the biscuit mixture with the sugar.

Suitable for vegetarians. Vegans should use vegan baking margarine and a non-dairy milk.

Cheese and Seed Oatcakes

Quintessentially Scottish, these savoury biscuits are traditionally very plain, but here they are flavoured with Parmesan and sesame seeds. They are always made from oatmeal rather than rolled or flaked oats, which is essentially the groat (the inside of the oat minus its inedible husk).

MAKES 16

100g medium oatmeal
100g self-raising wholemeal flour, plus extra for dusting
3 tbsp finely grated Parmesan cheese
3 tbsp sesame seeds
50g butter
75ml boiling water

1 Preheat the oven to 200°C/fan oven 180°C/gas 6. Line a baking sheet with baking paper. Put the oatmeal, flour, Parmesan and sesame seeds in a mixing bowl and stir to mix.
2 Melt the butter in a small saucepan, then add the boiling water. Pour over the dry ingredients, then, working quickly, mix everything together to make a soft dough; this will seem quite wet and sticky at first, but it will firm as the oatmeal absorbs the liquid.
3 Gently knead on a lightly floured work surface until smooth, then cut in half and roll out one piece to make a circle slightly smaller than 20cm; the dough should be about 3mm thick.
4 Cut into 8 triangles and carefully transfer them to the prepared baking sheet. Repeat with the remaining piece of dough.
5 Bake for 12–15 minutes until crisp, dry and lightly browned. Leave to cool on the baking sheet for 5 minutes, then transfer the oatcakes to a wire rack to cool completely. Store in an airtight tin for up to 2 weeks.

TIP

If you prefer, roll out the dough and stamp into rounds using a 7.5cm biscuit cutter. Knead the trimmings together, re-roll and stamp out more oatcakes.

VARIATION

Oatcakes can be flavoured in many ways: try adding 2 tsp caraway seeds or black or white poppy seeds to the mixture or ½ tsp dried thyme, for a change.

Suitable for vegetarians. Vegans should use a vegan Parmesan cheese substitute or add 1 tbsp nutritional yeast instead of the cheese and use a vegan baking margarine instead of the butter.

CONVERSION CHARTS

WEIGHT

Metric	Imperial
25g	1oz
50g	2oz
75g	3oz
100g	4oz
150g	5oz
175g	6oz
200g	7oz
225g	8oz
250g	9oz
300g	10oz
350g	12oz
400g	14oz
450g	1lb

OVEN TEMPERATURES

Celsius	Fahrenheit
110°C	225°F
120°C	250°F
140°C	275°F
150°C	300°F
160°C	325°F
170°C	340°F
180°C	350°F
190°C	375°F
200°C	400°F
220°C	425°F
230°C	450°F
240°C	475°F

LIQUIDS

Metric	Imperial	US cup
5ml	1 tsp	1 tsp
15ml	1 tbsp	1 tbsp
50ml	2fl oz	3 tbsp
60ml	2½fl oz	¼ cup
75ml	3fl oz	⅓ cup
100ml	4fl oz	scant ½ cup
125ml	4½ oz	½ cup
150ml	5fl oz	⅔ cup
200ml	7fl oz	scant 1 cup
250ml	9fl oz	1 cup
300ml	½ pint	1¼ cups
350ml	12fl oz	1 ½ cups
400ml	¾ pint	1¾ cups
500ml	17fl oz	2 cups
600ml	1 pt	2½ cups

Index

Abbreviations used in the index
(*GF*) gluten-free
(*V*) vegetarian
(*Vg*) vegan variation

A
aduki beans 70
afternoon snacks 17
agave syrup 29, 30, 31, 39, 43, 176, 177, 183
alfalfa seeds 70
All-Bran 172
almond butter 61
almond milk 156
almonds 20, 126, 142–3, 170, 171, 182
apple and blackberry base 143
apple and fennel salad 128, 129
apple purée 178, 179
apples 21, 32, 70
Apricot Spread (*V*) (*Vg*) 17, 27, 36–7
apricots 21, 112, 138–9 *see also* dried apricots
artichoke hearts 94
asparagus 116
Avocado and Watercress Dip (*V*) (*Vg*) 64–5, 74
avocados 21, 68, 83, 123
   chocolate mousse 156–7
   monounsaturated fats 157
   soluble and insoluble fibre 3

B
B-vitamins 11
bagel 'crisps' 53
baked beans 20
Baked Spanish Omelette (*V*) 80–1
Baked Vegetable Crisps (*V*) (*Vg*) 17, 18, 49, 66–7
baking 159
balanced diets 13
Banana and Date Loaf (*GF*) (*V*) 159, 170–1
banana ice cream 149
Banana Rice Pudding (*V*) (*Vg*) 133, 136–7
bananas 21, 33, 34–5, 136, 170–1
barley 4, 72–3
basmati rice 106–7, 130
beans 24–6
beansprouts 21, 60, 70, 71, 102, 114
Beef Jambalaya 91, 106–7
beetroot 21, 66
beneficial bacteria 6–7
black beans 176–7
black-eyed beans 84
black olives 76, 78, 122
blanched almonds 126
blood sugar levels 9
blueberries 33, 134
blueberry muffins 41
body mass index (BMI) 12
borlotti beans 56, 104
bowel motions 4–5
bran 15
bran cereal 172
bran flakes 20, 134, 180
Brazil nuts 20, 126–7
bread
   multi-grain 159, 162–3
   wholemeal 18, 20, 24

breadcrumbs 24, 62, 120, 124, 126
Breakfast Bars (V) (Vg) 27, 42–3
breakfast cereal 18, 27
breakfasts 17, 27
broccoli 21
brown basmati rice 106–7, 130
brown rice 18, 20, 136
brunches 27
brussels sprouts 21
burgers 124–5
buttermilk 166–7
Buttermilk Banana Pancakes (V) 27, 34–5
butternut squash 56, 113, 130, 144
Butternut Squash Cornbread (V) 166–7

C
cacao 148, 156
Cajun food 106
cancers 4, 9–11
canned fruit 152
cannellini beans 56
caramelised roasted onions 124
cardiovascular disease 11–12
Carrot and Coconut Cake (V) 17, 159, 174–5
carrots 21, 59, 64, 65, 174–5
cashew nuts 103
casseroling 92
Cauliflower and Chickpea Burgers (V) (Vg) 124–5
celeriac 56
celery sticks 21, 59, 64, 65
Cheddar and Watercress Scones (V) 159, 168–9
Cheddar cheese 76, 82, 116, 128, 168
Cheese and Potato Slice 128–9
Cheese and Seed Oatcakes (V) (Vg) 17, 49, 159, 186–7

Cheese-Topped Chicken and Mushroom Enchiladas 98–9
Cherry Bakewell Sponge (V) 142–3
cherry tomatoes 68, 78
chewing foods 12
chia seeds 15
chicken dishes
    Jambalaya 107
    Moroccan-style and chickpea casserole 92–3
    and mushroom and artichoke filo pie 94–5
    and mushroom enchiladas 98–9
    pan roast with vegetables 96
Chicken Noodle Soup (Vg) 49, 54–5
Chicken Satay Wraps 17, 60–1
Chickpea Scotch Eggs (V) 62–3
chickpeas 18, 20, 64, 88, 92–3, 124–5, 130
children 19
Chinese leaves 86
Chinese-Spiced Duck and Kumquats 91, 102–3
Chocolate and Avocado Mousse (V) (Vg) 17, 156–7
Chocolate and Coconut Ice Cream (V) (Vg) 148–9
Chocolate Chunk Black-Bean Brownies (GF) (V) (Vg) 159, 176–7
cholesterol 8, 11–12
chorizo sausages 106
Chunky Vegetable and Lentil Soup (V) (Vg) 49, 50–1
Classic Kimchi (V) (Vg) 86–7
Classic Minestrone (V) (Vg) 56–7
cocoa powder 148, 156, 176
coconut flakes 33, 137
coconut milk 140, 148–9, 156
coconut oil 176

cod 118–19
coleslaw 79, 88, 128
colons 6, 7
constipation 4–5, 7–8, 14
conversion charts 188–9
coriander 60, 62, 74, 88, 92
cornbread 167
cottage pie 108–9
couscous 17, 18, 20, 68, 92, 110–11, 112
cranberries 72–3
cream cheese 120
cream cheese frosting 175
Creamy Chicken, Mushroom and Artichoke Filo Pie 94–5
Crunchy Granola Cereal (V) (Vg) 27, 28–9
custard (V) (Vg) 138, 139

D
dairy products 8
dark chocolate 33, 156, 176, 177
date and walnut sponges 141
date syrup 23, 32, 33, 34–5
dates 21, 140, 148, 170
dehydration 14
desiccated coconut 20, 28, 174
dessert yogurt 150–1
desserts 133
Digestive Biscuits (V) (Vg) 17, 184–5
Dijon mustard dressing 122–3
dinner 17
Dips and Dippers (V) (Vg) 64
diverticulosis 7
dried apricots 21, 36–7, 42, 45, 84, 92, 151 see also apricots
dried bananas 136
dried dates 148
Dried Fruit Compote (V) (Vg) 38–9
dried fruits 18, 38

dried peaches 150–1
dried prunes 21, 112, 151
dried tropical fruit mix 172, 173
dry sherry 60, 114
duck 102–3
Duck and Mixed Mushroom Risotto 104–5
'dysbiosis' 6

E
egg custard 116–17
egg noodles 54
Eggs Benedict 46–7
endosperm 15
English muffins 46, 78

F
fennel 128, 129
Feta, Black-Eyed Bean and Potato Parcels (V) 84–5
fibre 1
  boosting intake 18
  daily intake 13–14, 19
  and fluids 14
  health and well-being 4–12
fibre-rich foods 6–7, 14–16, 20–1
figs 21, 154–5
filo pastry 84–5, 94–5
fish dishes see seafood
five-spice powder 102
flageolet beans 52
flaked almonds 142–3, 147
flax seeds (linseeds) 11, 15, 20, 32, 170, 176
focaccia 164–5
food labelling regulations 19
framboise 146
free radicals 10–11
Fresh Fig Compote (V) (Vg) 154–5
Fresh Tuna Niçoise 122–3
frozen yogurt 146

fruit jelly 152–3
fruits
  cancers 10
  fibre-rich foods 15, 18, 21
  five-a-day portions 16
  frozen and tinned 44
  insoluble fibre *3*
  soluble fibre *4*
full English breakfasts 27

G
gallbladder and gallstones 8–9
gelatine 152
germ 15
ginger 60, 86
Glazed Cod with Fresh Tomato
  Dressing 118–19
glucosinolates *10*
gluten-free diet (*GF*) 159
Goat's Cheese and Lentil Nut Loaf
  126–7
gochugaru (Korean chilli powder)
  86–7
grains 14, 20
granary bread 20
grapes 153
Greek-style yogurt 44, 46, 52, 146,
  154
green cabbage 50
green cardamom pods 138
green olives 78, 164
Green Pea and Flageolet Bean
  Soup (*V*) (*Vg*) 49, 52–3
groat 186
ground almonds 42, 142
ground cinnamon 40, 182
guacamole 74
gut bacteria 5–7

H
ham 46

hazelnuts 20, 28, 138, 174
heart attacks 4
high-calorie foods 12
high-density lipoproteins (HDL) 11
high-energy bars 42
hoisin sauce 114
honey 23, 30, 32–3, 34, 102–3, 112,
  162, 166, 170
Honey Biscuits 182–3
Honey Muffins 27, 40–1
hummus 64

I
indoles *10*
inflammatory diseases 4
insoluble fibre 3, *3*
irritable bowel syndrome (IBS) 7–8

J
Jambalaya 106–7

K
kidney beans 20
Kimchi 86–7
kiwi fruit 21
kumquats 102–3

L
lactose 8
lamb 109, 110
Lamb Tagine 17, 112–13
leafy vegetables *3*
lemon and ginger teabags 39
lentils (green) 20, 70
lentils (red split) 20, 50, 108, 126
Lighter Nachos 74–5
lignans 11
lime juice 60, 64, 65, 72, 74, 82,
  134, 135
lime zest 69, 82, 134, 135
losing weight 12–13

low-density lipoproteins (LDL) 11
Lower-Fat Eggs Benedict 46–7
Lower-Fat Hummus *(V) (Vg)* 49,
    64–5
lunch 17
lunchtime wraps 98 *see also*
    tortilla wraps
lycopene *10*

M
magnesium 5
main meals 91
maize *3*
mandolin 66
mango 33, 153
maple syrup 34, 140, 156
marinating meat 110
mascarpone cheese 134, 135
meal planning 17
meat dishes
    Beef Jambalaya 91, 106–7
    Cottage Pie 108–9
    Lamb Tagine 17, 112–13
    Stir-Fried Pork 114–15
Mediterranean Lamb and
    Vegetable Kebabs 91, 110–11
Medjool dates 23, 148
Melting-Middle Fishcakes 120–1
mid-morning snacks 17
milk 8, 30
minced beef 108
minestrone *(V) (Vg)* 56–7
Mini Pizza Grills 78–9
Minted Yogurt 52–3, 92
mixed bean salad 99
monounsaturated fats 11–12, 157
Monterey Jack cheese 82
Moroccan-Style Chicken and
    Chickpea Casserole 91, 92–3
mozzarella cheese 74, 78
muesli 162

muffins 40–1, 46, 78
Multi-Grain Bread 159, 162–3
mung beans 70
mushrooms 94–5, 98, 104–5, 128

N
naan breads 130, 131
nachos 74
natural yogurt 32, 64, 88
No-Bake Blueberry Cheesecake
    (V) 133, 134–5
nuts 15, 18, 20–1, 138

O
Oat and Apple Cookies *(V)* 159,
    178–9
oat bran 20, 31, 184
Oat Bran and Honey Muffins *(V)*
    27, 40–1
oatcakes 186–7
oatmeal 150, 184, 186
oats *4*, 20, 27, 138
Oaty Apricot Crumble *(V) (Vg)* 97,
    133, 138–9
obesity 12
olive oil 84, 85
olive-oil flatbread 164
omega-3 fat 15
One-Pan Roast Chicken with
    Vegetables 96–7
orange juice 68, 72, 150, 152
orange liqueur 150
orange zest 68
oranges 21, 152–3
Oriental Sprouted Salad *(V) (Vg)*
    70–1
osteoporosis 4
oven-baked crisps 66
Overnight Oats *(V) (Vg)* 17, 27, 32–3
overweight 11, 12
oxidation 11

P
pak choi 102, 103
para-coumaric acid *10*
Parmesan cheese 56, 186
passata 58
pasta 18, 56, 100 *see also* spaghetti
pastry 144–5
peach purée 150–1
peach schnapps 150
peaches 21
Peaches and Cream Winter Fool
    (V) 150–1
peanut butter 20, 60, 61, 180–1
Peanut Butter Cookies 180–1
peanuts 20, 42, 126–7
Pear and Raspberry Smoothie *(V)*
    (Vg) 44–5
pearl barley 72, 73
pears 21, 72
peas 21, 52–3, 54, 80, 105
pecan nuts 72, 171, 182
Pecorino cheese 116, 117
pepperoni salami stick 78
pesto 58
phytates 13
phytochemicals 6, 10
phytoestrogens *10*
pies 94
pine nuts 169
Pineapple and Orange Jelly 152–3
pinto beans 82
pitta bread 20, 88
pizzas 76–9
plum tomatoes 76, 122
poaching eggs 46
polenta (cornmeal) 166
poppy seeds 84, 160
porcini mushrooms 104
pork 114
porridge 20, 30–1
porridge (rolled) oats 28, 32–3, 42

pot barley 72
potatoes 7, 8, 21, 84
    cottage pie 108–9
    crisps 66–7
    fishcakes 120–1
    omelettes 80
    soups 52, 56–7
prawns 68, 107
prunes 21, 112, 151
puddings and bakes 142
pulses 15, 24–6
    boosting fibre intake 18
    dips 64
    fibre-rich foods 14, 20
    insoluble fibre 3
    soaking and cooking 25–6
    soluble fibre 4
    sprouting 70–1
Pumpkin Pie *(V)* 144–5
pumpkin seeds 21, 162
pumpkin squash 56, 144

Q
quiche 116–17
quinoa 31, 88
Quinoa Berry Porridge *(V) (Vg)* 30–1
Quinoa Falafels in Wholemeal
    Pittas *(V) (Vg)* 88–90
quinoa flakes 30, 31

R
radishes 70, 86
raisin and coconut cookies 179
raisins 21, 42, 174
rapeseed oil 28, 29
ras-el-hanout 112, 113
raspberries 21, 44, 146
Raspberry and Rose Frozen
    Yogurt *(V)* 133, 146–7
Re-Fried Bean Burritos with
    Fresh Tomato Salsa *(V)* 82

red kidney beans 18, 25, 74, 106
red lentils 50, 108, 126
red onions 74
red peppers 58, 78, 86
redcurrant jelly 134, 135
refined carbohydrates 9
resistant starch 7
rheumatoid arthritis 4
rice
    brown basmati rice 106–7, 130
    brown rice 18, 20, 136
    insoluble fibre 3
    white rice 104, 136
rice pudding 136–7
rice wine 114
rice wine vinegar 70
risottos 104
Roasted Red Pepper and Tomato
    Soup (V) (Vg) 49, 58–9
roasting cauliflower 124
roasting peppers 58
rolled oats 28, 32–3, 42
root vegetables 4
rosewater 146
'roughage' 1
rye 4
rye bread 20
rye flour 162, 163

S
salads 49
    Fresh Tuna Niçoise 122–3
    mixed bean salad 99
    Oriental Sprouted Salad (V)
        (Vg) 70–1
    Turkey and Cranberry Salad
        with Barley 72–3
    Warm Prawn, Avocado and
        Wholewheat Couscous Salad
        68–9
salmon 116–17

satay sauce 60
Scotch Eggs (V) 62–3
seafood
    cod 118–19
    prawns 68–9, 107
    salmon 116–17
    tuna 120–1, 122–3
seeds 15, 20–1, 138
serotonin 5–6
sesame oil 70
sesame seeds 21, 28, 42, 70, 103,
    116, 160, 186
shallots 102, 103
shepherd's pie 109
short-chain fatty acids 4, 6
smart shopping 19
Smoked Salmon and Asparagus
    Quiche with a Spelt and
    Sesame Crust 116–17
snacks 18, 49
soluble fibre 3, 4, 8, 9
soups 49
    Chicken Noodle 54–5
    Green Pea and Flageolet Bean
        Soup 52–3
    Minestrone 56–7
    Roasted Red Pepper and
        Tomato Soup 58–9
    Vegetable and Lentil Soup 50–1
soy sauce 60, 70, 102
spaghetti 20, 57, 100 see also pasta
Spanish Omelette (V) 80–1
spelt 116, 182
spiralised courgetti 100
spring greens 21
spring onions 21, 63, 86
sprouted pulses 70, 71
Sticky Toffee Puddings (V) 133,
    140–1
stir-fries 114
strawberries 33

strokes 4, 11–12

strong white bread flour 160, 162–3, 164–5

strong wholemeal bread flour 164

sultanas 21, 92

Sun-Dried Tomato and Olive Focaccia *(V) (Vg)* 159, 164–5

sun-dried tomato paste 78

sun-dried tomatoes 64, 98, 111, 164

sunflower seeds 21, 29, 138, 162

swede 56, 108

Sweet and Spicy Stir-Fried Pork 114–15

Sweet Potato Bread Rolls *(V)* 159, 160–1

sweet potatoes 21, 66

sweetcorn 21, 54, 120

symbiosis 6

T

tagines 112

tahini 64

terpenes *10*

tikka masala curry paste 130

toasted nuts and seeds 31

tofu 55

tomato dressing 118–19

tomato salsa 74, 82

tomato sauce 100–1

tomatoes 21, 81

Tortilla Chips *(V) (Vg)* 49, 66–7

tortilla wraps 20, 60, 74, 82–3, 98–9

triglycerides 11

Tropical Fruit Malt Teabread *(V) (Vg)* 172–3

tuna 120, 122

Turkey and Cranberry Salad with Barley 72–3

Turkey Meatballs in Tomato Sauce 100–1

type-1 diabetes 9

type-2 diabetes 4, 9

Tzatziki 110–11, 124

U

ultra-high fibre 'diet' products 13

Updated Cottage Pie 108–9

Upside-Down Pizza *(V)* 76–7

V

vanilla extract 36, 140, 148, 156

vanilla pods 38–9, 154–5

vegan dishes *(Vg)* 15, 91

vegetable crisps *(V) (Vg)* 66–7

vegetable crudités 64, 65

vegetable sauces 118

Vegetable Tikka Masala *(V) (Vg)* 130–1

vegetables
    cancers 10
    dips 64
    fibre-rich foods 15, 18, 21
    five-a-day portions 16

vegetarian burgers *(V)* 124–5

vegetarian curry *(V)* 130–1

vegetarian dishes *(V)* 15, 91

vine vegetables *4*

W

walnut oil 68

walnuts 15, 21, 72, 171, 182

Warm Prawn, Avocado and Wholewheat Couscous Salad 68–9

water chestnuts 102

watercress 64–5, 168

weight loss 12–13

wheat *3*

wheat bran 13

wheatgerm 20, 31, 44, 162, 164

white flour 144, 168, 174

white rice 104, 136
white wine vinegar 70
whole grains 11, 15
wholegrain foods 18
wholemeal bread 18, 20
wholemeal breadcrumbs 24, 62,
    120, 124, 126
wholemeal flour
    cookies 178
    Digestive Biscuits 184
    multi-grain bread 162
    Oat Bran and Honey Muffins 40
    pancakes 34
    pastry 144
    pizza 76–7
    puddings 140
    scones 168
wholemeal muffins 46, 78
wholemeal pitta bread 20, 88
wholemeal spaghetti 20, 57, 100

Wholemeal Spelt and Honey
    Biscuits *(V) (Vg)* 159, 182–3
wholemeal spelt flour 116, 182
wholemeal tortilla wraps 20, 60,
    74, 82–3, 98–9
wholewheat breakfast cereal 18, 27
wholewheat couscous 17, 18, 20,
    68, 92, 110–11, 112
wholewheat egg noodles 54
wholewheat naan breads 130, 131
wholewheat pasta 18, 56, 100
wholewheat spaghetti 57, 100
World Cancer Research Fund 9–
    10

Y
yeast 88, 160
yellow peppers 76, 78
yellow polenta (cornmeal) 166
yogurt hollandaise 46